Neurological Drugs

Celebrating 50 Years

Passion, Quality and Innovation in Healthcare Publishing

Neurological Drugs

Vikas Dhikav
MBBS, MD (3 years, AIIMS), PhD (Neurology), DSc (Honorary)
Fellowship in Cognitive Neurology
Fellowship in Clinical Neuropsychopharmacology
Honorary Professor
International School of Medicine
International University of Kyrgyzstan (ISM-IUK)
Bishkek, Kyrgyzstan
Former Visiting Faculty
Southern Medical University
Jinan Medical University, Dali University
Wuhan, Nanchang and Luzhou Universities
People Republic of China
Consultant
Indian Council of Medical Research
Department of Health Research
Ministry of Health and Family Welfare
Government of India, New Delhi, India

Forewords
Professor (Dr) Balram Bhargava
KS Anand

JAYPEE BROTHERS MEDICAL PUBLISHERS
The Health Sciences Publisher
New Delhi | London | Panama

Jaypee Brothers Medical Publishers (P) Ltd

Headquarters

Jaypee Brothers Medical Publishers (P) Ltd
4838/24, Ansari Road, Daryaganj
New Delhi 110 002, India
Phone: +91-11-43574357
Fax: +91-11-43574314
E-mail: jaypee@jaypeebrothers.com

Overseas Offices

JP Medical Ltd
83 Victoria Street, London
SW1H 0HW (UK)
Phone: +44 20 3170 8910
Fax: +44 (0)20 3008 6180
E-mail: info@jpmedpub.com

Jaypee-Highlights Medical Publishers Inc
City of Knowledge, Bld. 235, 2nd Floor
Clayton, Panama City, Panama
Phone: +1 507-301-0496
Fax: +1 507-301-0499
E-mail: cservice@jphmedical.com

Jaypee Brothers Medical Publishers (P) Ltd
Bhotahity, Kathmandu, Nepal
Phone: +977-9741283608
E-mail: kathmandu@jaypeebrothers.com

Website: www.jaypeebrothers.com
Website: www.jaypeedigital.com

Neurological Drugs

First Edition: **2019**

ISBN 978-93-5270-900-7

Printed at Rajkamal Electric Press, Plot No. 2, Phase-IV, Kundli, Haryana.

Dedicated to

Little angel daughters, Priyanshi and Princi
and beloved wife, Meenakshi Dhikav

Foreword

सत्यमेव जयते

प्रोफेसर (डा.) बलराम भार्गव, पदम श्री
एमडी, डीएम, एफआरसीपी (जी.), एफआरसीपी (ई.),
एफएसीसी, एफएएचए, एफएएमएस, एफएनएएससी, एफएएससी
सचिव, भारत सरकार
स्वास्थ्य अनुसंधान विभाग
स्वास्थ्य एवं परिवार कल्याण मंत्रालय एवं
महानिदेशक, आई सी एम आर

Prof. (Dr.) Balram Bhargava, Padma Shri
MD, DM, FRCP (Glasg.), FRCP (Edin.),
FACC, FAHA, FAMS, FNASc, FASc
Secretary to the Government of India
Department of Health Research
Ministry of Health & Family Welfare &
Director-General, ICMR

भारतीय आयुर्विज्ञान अनुसंधान परिषद
स्वास्थ्य अनुसंधान विभाग
स्वास्थ्य एवं परिवार कल्याण मंत्रालय
वी. रामलिंगस्वामी भवन, अंसारी नगर,
नई दिल्ली– 110029 (भारत)

Indian Council of Medical Research
Department of Health Research
Ministry of Health & Family Welfare
V. Ramalingaswami Bhawan, Ansari Nagar
New Delhi – 110029 (INDIA)

Professional information on drugs used in neurological disorders is limited in Indian context. *Neurological Drugs* is an attempt to update postgraduates and practicing doctors about the neurological drug therapy.

The author has attempted to include several topics in this small volume, yet the book may be concise but is comprehensive. The presentation is lucid and the language is simple.

The author needs to be congratulated for the excellent efforts in the direction of brining this book. I hope the book will be very useful for the intended audience and for anyone who is interested in the practice of neurology/psychiatry/neuropsychiatry.

(Balram Bhargava)

Foreword

[illegible]

(Balram Bhargava)

Foreword

Government of India

Neurological drugs is a unique compilation of Neurology Drug Reference in India. In this small but comprehensive book, the author has been able to successfully combine the Art and Science used in treatment of Neurological Disorders. This book is the first of its kind for Indian subcontinent and will go a long way in providing first hand knowledge to budding physicians, neurologists and psychiatrists alike.

KS Anand
DM (Neuro) MNAMS (Neuro) FIAN FAMS FRCP (London)
FICP FIAMS FIMSA FIACM MBA
Fellowship in Movement Disorders (USA) and
Neurorehabilitation (VMMC)
Member, American Academy of Neurology
Professor of Neurology
Senior Consultant Neurologist and Head
Department of Neurology
Postgraduate Institute of Medical Education and
Research, Chandigarh and
Dr Ram Manohar Lohia Hospital
New Delhi, India

Preface

Neurological Drugs is perceived as one of the most difficult topics during entire medical curriculum. In the MBBS, when the foundation for being the medical doctor is being laid; this topic is either not taught or is taught at a superficial level.

In MD, when the Master Degree training program is in full flow, not enough attention is given to this. Additionally, no lectures are held for MD students assuming this would have been done at MBBS level.

At DM level, when one is expected to have an astute understanding of neuropharmacology; clinical details and follow-up consume much of the time. Again this topic takes back seat, at the final time, when it should have been finally dealt. Hence, hardly any time is left for trainee to get hold of this valuable subject. The present book is aimed at fulfilling these gaps.

One of the challenges while writing this book was that the available information comes from the west which may not be relevant. For example, dose requirements may be different, and pharmacokinetic and pharmacodynamic differences may be prominent in some cases. Western patients may have faster metabolic speed leading to smaller blood levels at lower doses (which may be appropriate in Asian patients). Hence, it is important to have Indian reference dose range that our hardworking clinicians have been using since ages. Unfortunately, in the absence of published data, it becomes difficult to produce a unifying source for the same. However, the present book can be a starting point and with passage of time such details will emerge and the growth of the book can be proportional.

Vikas Dhikav

Acknowledgments

I wish to acknowledge the help of Memory Clinic, Department of Neurology, Postgraduate Institute of Medical Education and Research, Chandigarh and Dr Ram Manohar Lohia Hospital, New Delhi, India for offering generous support in writing this book.

I would like to thank Shri Jitendar P Vij (Group Chairman), Mr Ankit Vij (Managing Director), Ms Chetna Malhotra Vohra (Associate Director—Content Strategy), Ms Prerna Bajaj (Development Editor), and all the staff of M/s Jaypee Brothers Medical Publishers, New Delhi, India, for their efforts and input enabling timely publication of the book.

Vikas Dhikav
New Delhi, India
vikasdhikav@hotmail.com

Contents

CHAPTER

1

Drugs in Neurological Practice

INTRODUCTION

Rita Levi-Montalcini (1986 Nobel Prize in Medicine) said "in the 19th century and at the beginning of the 20th century, brain research belonged to many different areas that differed in methodology and targets: the morphological, the physiological, and the psychological. Due to prolonged aging, neurodevelopmental disorders are growing and a much deeper knowledge of the brain is necessary". Drugs can play an important role in diagnosis, treatment, or prevention of neurological disorders.

As per World Health Organization, neurological disorders are one of the greatest threats to mankind. Drug therapy is cornerstone of the treatment.

NEUROLOGICAL DRUGS: CHALLENGES AND OPPORTUNITIES

Parkinson disease is a common neurodegenerative disease. The drug treatment is quite effective and Levodopa is the most effective drug treatment. However, its chronic use is associated with dyskinesia, motor fluctuations, and hallucinations.[1] Hence, in neurology, like in any other clinical specialty, there is a need to develop treatment strategies that allow stratification of therapies to optimize efficacy and minimize toxicity.[2] Patients always have expectations from the doctors, especially in neurology as the nature of disease/s may be protracted (Fig. 1.1).

Drug-induced neurologic conditions may result from single-agent drug regimens, but they are more likely to occur when multiple agents that confer risk are administered concomitantly. Educating patients about these risks and remaining vigilant in clinical investigations of unusual adverse effects are key elements to increasing the safety of drug management.[3]

Newer drugs may be safe but may not always be effective so one would have to manage drug therapy carefully.[4]

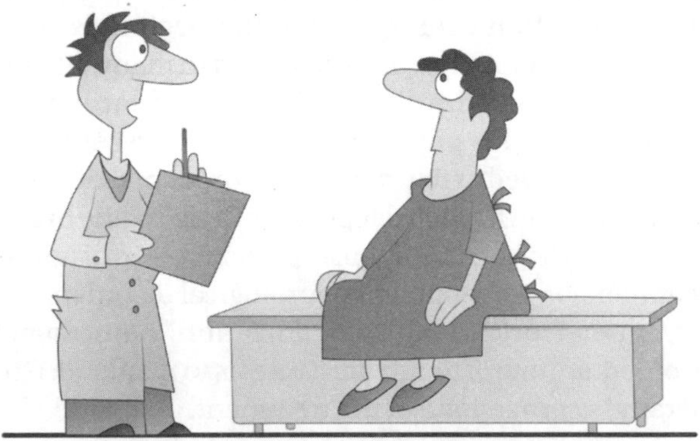

"The only diet shake I recommend is the shake your body makes when you exercise"

Fig. 1.1: Patients often have unrealistic expectations and may land up after having been seen by many doctors. A neurologist is always confronted with such patients and a combination of counseling, assurance, and delicate handling avoiding false reassurances helps.

CONCLUSION

Doctors often get puzzling neurological problems in general practice for many of which there is no effective medical treatment. However, effective drugs are available for many of the most common conditions like headache, neuralgia, seizure disorders, movement disorders, facial palsy, dementias, cerebrovascular accidents, and meningitis etc. One of the most effective ways to use proper medications is to ensure proper selection based upon pharmacological profile of drugs.

REFERENCES

1. Jankovic J. Complications and limitations of drug therapy for Parkinson's disease. Neurology. 2000;55(12 Suppl 6):S2-6.
2. Chan A, Pirmohamed M, Comabella M. Pharmacogenomics in neurology: current state and future steps. Ann Neurol. 2011;70(5):684-97.
3. Medscape. (2017). Drug-induced neurologic conditions. [online] Available from www.medscape.com/viewarticle/822551. [Accessed May, 2018].
4. Kane JM. Newer antipsychotic drugs. A review of their pharmacology and therapeutic potential. Drugs. 1993;46(4):585-93.

CHAPTER

2

Neural Basis of Neurological Disorders

NEUROLOGICAL DISORDERS AT A GLANCE

Diseases in neurology range from minor functional to severe, life-threatening diseases with structural or neuroanatomical basis (Box 2.1).[1]

It is indeed one of the first thing in neurology to be able to localize and typify the nature of disease for successful treatment.

Malignant Disorders

Cancer[2] is basically a mass of cells whose growth is uncontrolled and that serve no useful function. Malignant

Box 2.1: Broad category of neurological diseases.

- *Functional disorders*:
  - For example, primary headaches
- Malignant disorders
- Seizure disorders
- Cerebrovascular accidents
- Disorders of development
- Degenerative disorders.

tumor on the other hand is a cancerous tumor, and lacks distinct border and may metastasize. This is the most serious type of cancer.

Glioma is a cancerous brain tumor composed of one of several types of glial cells. This is usually detected late and is hard to treat as well.

However, not all tumors in the brain are not malignant; some are benign tumors also, e.g. a noncancerous tumor; has a distinct border and cannot metastasize. Meningioma is a benign brain tumor composed of the cells that constitute the meninges.

There >100 central nervous system tumors and are classified as per WHO's classification depending upon whether the tumor is benign or malignant. Depending upon rate of growth, grading is given, e.g. Grade I (least malignant) to Grade IV (most malignant). Common central nervous system tumors include acoustic neuroma, astrocytoma, chordoma, lymphoma, craniopharyngioma, brainstem, glioma, ependymoma, mixed glioma, optic nerve glioma, medulloblastoma, meningioma, metastatic tumors, oligodendroglioma, pituitary tumors, neuroectodermal tumors and schwannoma etc. tumors like brainstem glioma, craniopharyngioma, ependymoma, medulloblastoma and neuroectodermal tumors are more common in children.

Treatment involves surgery whether conventional or gamma knife or conservative such as radiotherapy, chemotherapy, or symptomatic therapies.

Seizures[3]

Seizures are recurrent convulsions. Partial seizures do not involve the whole brain. Generalized seizures on the other hand involves the entire brain and are widespread. Seizures could be of many types (Box 2.2).

Box 2.2: Types of seizures.

Partial seizures:
- Simple
- Complex.

Generalized seizures:
- *Grand mal*—Generalized, tonic/clonic
- Absence (petit mal).

Box 2.3: Causes of seizures.

- Head injury
- Stroke
- Developmental abnormalities
- Tumor
- Febrile seizures
- Fever
- Alcohol or barbiturate withdrawal
- Genetic factors.

Antiepileptic drugs increase inhibitory mechanisms and reduce excitatory pathways (Box 2.3). They increase Cl^- influx or decrease gamma-aminobutyric acid (GABA) metabolism and provide cellular inhibition. Block of sodium channels or antagonist of α-amino-3-hydroxy-5-methyl-4-isoxazolepropionic acid (AMPA)/N-methyl-D-aspartate (NMDA) mechanisms may also help by reducing excitability of neurons.

Cerebrovascular Accidents[4]

Block in the blood vessels feeding the brain or bleeding can cause cerebrovascular accident or stroke. It can be:

- *Hemorrhagic stroke* that occurs due to rupture of a cerebral blood vessel.
- *Clot leading to stroke (thrombotic stroke)*: This can be obstructive stroke that occurs due to occlusion of a blood vessel and is the most common type. This can

be due to either thrombus—blood clot that forms within a blood vessel or embolus—piece of material that forms in one part of the vascular system, breaks off, and carried by bloodstream until it reaches a smaller artery.

Transient ischemic attack (TIA) is temporary or focal loss of neurologic function. It is caused by ischemia of one of the blood vessels present in the vascular territories of the brain. Microemboli with temporary blockage of blood flow could be the reasons behind this. TIA lasts for less than 24 hours and often less than 15 minutes or so. Importantly, most cases resolve within 3 hours. This could however be the warning sign of progressive cerebrovascular disease and a stroke may recur.

Clinically, sudden numbness or weakness of face, arms, or legs, especially on one side of the body or sudden confusion or trouble speaking or understanding speech could be the presenting features. Additionally, sudden trouble seeing in one or both eyes or sudden trouble walking, dizziness, or loss of balance or coordination could be clinical features. Sudden severe headache with no known cause could indicate subarachnoid bleed.

Ischemic cascade sets off upon interruption of blood supply to brain. Series of metabolic events such as inadequate ATP adenosine triphosphate production, loss of ion homeostasis, release of excitatory amino acids and increase in glutamate production leading to free radical formation and cell death occur. Border zone exists with a reversible area that surrounds the core ischemic area in which there is reduced blood flow but which can be restored with in about 3 hours.

Brain gets a large chunk of blood supply, i.e. 20% of cardiac output about 1000 mL/min. More than 30 second, interruption of blood supply can cause neurologic metabolism alteration and metabolism stops in 2 minutes leading to brain cell death < 5 minutes.

Atherosclerosis is the major cause of cerebrovascular accidents (Thrombotic type). Thrombus formation and emboli development is dependent upon abnormal filtration of lipids in the intimal layer of the arterial wall. Plaque develops at locations of increased turbulence of blood, e.g. bifurcations of vessels leading to increased turbulence of blood or a tortuous area. Calcified plaques rupture or fissure are additional causes. Platelets and fibrin adhere to the plaque. Narrowing or blockage of an artery by thrombus or emboli could be additional. Cerebral infarction occurs when the blocked artery with blood supply cuts off beyond the point of blockage.

Thrombotic stroke needs clot busting (thrombolytic therapy) within 3 hours of onset while hemorrhagic stroke treatment is mainly symptomatic.

Metabolic Disorders[5]

Tay-Sachs disease is a metabolic "storage" disease. One or more enzymes are missing, waste products cannot be destroyed by lysosomes accumulation.[5]

Lysosomes get larger, cells get larger, and brain swells.

Symptoms begin around 4 months and include exaggerated startle response, listlessness, irritability, spasticity, seizures, dementia, and death.

Enzyme replacement therapy is treatment of choice but is not widely available for treatment of lysosomal storage diseases.

Genetic Diseases[6]

Trisomy 21 is a common one caused by a nondisjunction event. A gamete (a sperm or egg cell) is produced with an extra copy of chromosome 21. Nondisjunction is the failure of chromosome pairs to separate properly during cell division. The result of this error is a cell with an imbalance of chromosomes.

There is no known cure but early detection and treating complications can be done.

Degenerative Diseases[7,8]

Transmissible spongiform encephalopathies are an uncommon degenerative disease. It is a contagious brain disease whose degenerative process gives the brain a sponge-like appearance. Creutzfeldt-Jakob disease (CJD), fatal familial insomnia, kuru (humans), and scrapie (sheep) are types. These are caused by prions. Prions are protein that can exist in two forms that differ only in their three-dimensional (3D) shape.

Degenerative diseases of this nature can be familial, sporadic, and acquired including iatrogenic.

There is no known cure for CJD but drugs like antiviral agents, interferons, and corticosteroids have been tried.

Movement Disorders[9]

Parkinson's disease is the most common movement disorder encountered clinically. It is a disease caused by degeneration of the nigrostriatal system—the dopamine-secreting neurons of the substantia nigra [send axons to basal ganglia (BG)]. Lewy body—abnormal circular structures with a dense core consisting of alpha-synuclein (SNCA) protein (presynaptic protein); found in dopaminergic nigrostriatal neurons of Parkinson's patients.

Gene mutations, e.g. mutation on chromosome 4 play an important role. Genes that code for SNCA—located in presynaptic terminal of dopamine cells. Toxic gain of function may occur.

Abnormal SNCA becomes misfolded, forms aggregations—make up Lewy bodies. Mutation on chromosome 6—produces an abnormal Parkin protein. Normal Parkin plays a role in trafficking defective/misfolded proteins to proteasomes for destruction (recycling). Defective Parkin allows abnormally high levels of defective proteins to accumulate in dopaminergic neurons. Fail to ubiquitinate abnormal proteins. Ubiquitination targets the abnormal proteins for destruction by the proteasomes and this may kill the cell.

Parkinson's disease affects 1% of people over 65. The common symptoms are given here in Box 2.4.

Parkinson's disease is treating by resetting balance between cholinergic and dopaminergic pathways.

Huntington's Disease[9]

This is not an uncommon disease and occurs due to degeneration of caudate nucleus and putamen. Clinically, it presents as uncontrollable movements, jerky limb movements. The disease is progressive, and cognitive and emotional changes can occur. Death usually occurs within 10–15 years. The disease can affect both men and women.

Huntington's disease (HD) is caused by an autosomal dominant mutation in either of an individual's two copies of a gene called *huntingtin (htt)*, which means any child of an affected person typically has a 50% chance of inheriting the disease.

Physical symptoms of HD can begin at any age from infancy to old age, but usually begin between 35 years and 44 years of age. Some cases starting in teen age can have akinetic-rigid syndrome; they progress faster and vary slightly.

Box 2.4: Symptoms of Parkinson's disease.

- Muscular rigidity
- Slowness of movement
- Resting tremor
- Postural instability
- Difficulties with handwriting or making facial expressions.

The disease is associated with dominant gene on chromosome 4. Gene that codes the *htt* protein is associated with repeated sequence of bases that code for the amino acid glutamine.

Abnormal *htt* becomes misfolded and forms aggregates in nucleus and accounts for cell death and apoptosis.

Dopaminergic excess of HD is treated by antidopaminergic drugs (D2 blockers, e.g. haloperidol).

Dementia[10]

This is the most common neurodegenerative brain disorder of unknown origin among aged and causes progressive memory loss, motor deficits, and death. About 10% of the population over 65 years old and 50% of the population over 85 years old.[10]

It starts with misplacing things and losing the ability to retrace steps. Decreased or poor judgment can occur.

Severe degeneration of the hippocampus, entorhinal cortex and neocortex (prefrontal and temporal association areas), locus coeruleus, and raphe nucleus can occur. Memory loss may disrupt daily life if dementia supervenes. Challenges in planning or solving problems can appear. One would encounter difficulty in completing familiar tasks at home, at work, or at leisure. Confusion with time or place can appear with passage of time. Trouble in understanding visual images and spatial relationships also develops.

One may start to withdraw from work or social activities. Changes in mood and personality may occur as well. Amyloid plaque—extracellular deposit containing a dense core of β-amyloid protein surrounded by degenerating axons and dendrites and activated microglia and reactive astrocytes.

Neurofibrillary tangle—a dying neuron containing intracellular accumulations of abnormally phosphorylated tau-protein filaments that formerly served as the cell's internal skeleton is the hallmark of Alzheimer's disease.

The major form of dementia, e.g. Alzheimer's disease involves reduced function of acetylcholine in various brain areas; hence the treatment involves anticholinesterases.

Multiple Sclerosis[11]

Autoimmune demyelinating disease with sclerotic plaques. It is an autoimmune disease which is when the body starts to destroy itself. It is a life-long disease with no cure but the disease can be suppressed.

In multiple sclerosis (MS), the body attacks and destroys the fatty tissue called myelin that insulates an axon/nerve, and is called demyelination (Fig. 2.1). If damage is severe, it can also destroy the nerve/axon itself. MS affects the central nervous system and inflames the white matter in the brain which creates plaques.

Treatment involves beta interferons and monoclonal antibodies like ocrelizumab, natalizumab, alemtuzumab, etc. Glatiramer acetate, dimethyl fumarate, and fingolimod are immunomodulators used.

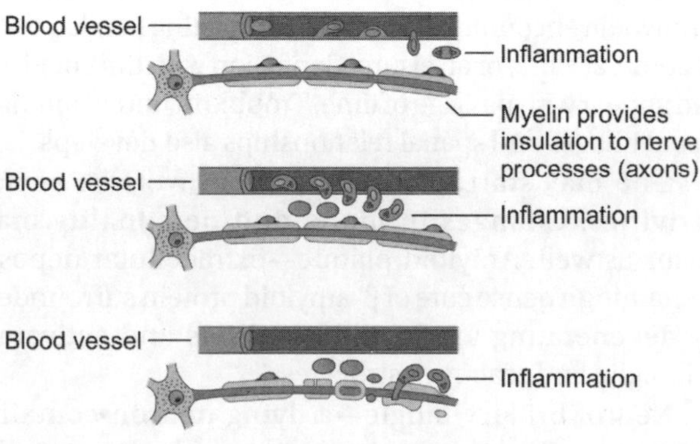

Fig. 2.1: Basically, multiple sclerosis (MS) is a chronic inflammatory demyelinating disease of the brain and spinal cord.

Myasthenia Gravis[12]

This is an acquired autoimmune disorder, clinically characterized by: weakness of skeletal muscles and fatigability on exertion. First clinical description was given in 1672 by Thomas Willis.

In myasthenia gravis, antibodies are directed toward the acetylcholine receptor at the neuromuscular junction of skeletal muscles. This results in decreased number of nicotinic acetylcholine receptors at the motor endplate. Also, reduced postsynaptic membrane folds and widened synaptic cleft can occur.

Drugs useful in myasthenia gravis inhibit the enzyme acetylcholinesterase and increase acetylcholine levels in synaptic cleft.

CONCLUSION

Neurological diseases include tumors, seizure disorders, cerebrovascular accidents, disorders of development and neurodegenerative disorders. Diabetes affects brain, spinal cord and nerves in several ways.

Malignancies consist of mass of cells whose growth is uncontrolled and that serves no useful function. Malignant tumors lack distinct borders and may metastasize. Benign tumor is a noncancerous tumor and has a distinct border and cannot metastasize. For example, glioma is a cancerous brain tumor composed of one of several types of glial cells and meningioma—a benign brain tumor composed of the cells that constitute the meninges.

Partial seizures do not involve the whole brain but generalized seizures involve the entire brain, and have widespread effect. Partial seizures are of two types: simple and complex. Grand mal seizures are generalized, tonic/clonic seizures while absence (Petit mal) seizures are generalized, with absence of abnormal movements/behavioral manifestations. Common causes of seizures include brain injury, stroke, developmental abnormalities, tumors and febrile seizures etc. A variety of anti-seizure drugs are used for treatment.

Hemorrhagic stroke involves rupture of a cerebral blood vessel and obstructive stroke which is more common is due to occlusion of a blood vessel. Thrombus is a blood clot that forms within a blood vessel but embolus is a piece of material that forms in one part of the vascular system, breaks off, carried by bloodstream until it reaches a smaller artery and causes infarction. Thrombolytic agents are mainstay of treatment.

Exposure to toxic chemicals during pregnancy, impair fetal development. Ingestion of alcohol or smoking during pregnancy or German measles can affect brain development. Additionally, inherited metabolic disorders, e.g. Phenylketonuria or Tay-Sachs disease could be seen.

REFERENCES

1. Probyn K, Bowers H, Mistry D, et al. Non-pharmacological self-management for people living with migraine or tension-type headache: a systematic review including analysis of intervention components. BMJ Open. 2017;7(8):e016670.
2. Huncharek M, Muscat J, Geschwind JF. Multi-drug versus single agent chemotherapy for high grade astrocytoma; results of a meta-analysis. Anticancer Res. 1998;18(6B):4693-7.
3. Ngugi AK, Bottomley C, Kleinschmidt I, et al. Estimation of the burden of active and life-time epilepsy: a meta-analytic approach. Epilepsia. 2010;51(5):883-90.
4. Guekht A, Vester J, Heiss WD, et al. Safety and efficacy of Cerebrolysin in motor function recovery after stroke: a meta-analysis of the CARS trials. Neurol Sci. 2017;38(10):1761-9.

5. Schoser B, Stewart A, Kanters S, et al. Survival and long-term outcomes in late-onset Pompe disease following alglucosidase alfa treatment: a systematic review and meta-analysis. J Neurol. 2017;264(4):621-30.
6. Lee NC, Chien YH, Hwu WL. A review of biomarkers for Alzheimer's disease in Down syndrome. Neurol Ther. 2017;6(Suppl 1):69-81.
7. Zhu ZG, Sun MX, Zhang WL, et al. The efficacy and safety of coenzyme Q10 in Parkinson's disease: a meta-analysis of randomized controlled trials. Neurol Sci. 2017;38(2):215-24.
8. Varges D, Manthey M, Heinemann U, et al. Doxycycline in early CJD: a double-blinded randomised phase II and observational study. J Neurol Neurosurg Psychiatry. 2017;88(2):119-25.
9. Squitieri F, de Yebenes JG. Profile of pridopidine and its potential in the treatment of Huntington disease: the evidence to date. Drug Des Devel Ther. 2015;9:5827-33.
10. Tan L, Tan L, Wang HF, et al. Efficacy and safety of atypical antipsychotic drug treatment for dementia: a systematic review and meta-analysis. Alzheimers Res Ther. 2015;7(1):20.
11. Ontaneda D, Fox RJ, Chataway J. Clinical trials in progressive multiple sclerosis: lessons learned and future perspectives. Lancet Neurol. 2015;14(2):208-23.
12. Melzer N, Ruck T, Fuhr P, et al. Clinical features, pathogenesis, and treatment of myasthenia gravis: a supplement to the Guidelines of the German Neurological Society. J Neurol. 2016;263(8):1473-94.

CHAPTER

3

Therapeutic Targets in Neuropharmacology

INTRODUCTION

Questions such as how do drugs act at cell surfaces of brain neurons to alter processes inside cells come to everyone's mind.

The key is what points in biochemical pathways are rate limiting and thus potential sites at which drugs act to alter pathways and become useful in neurological diseases?

One of the long-standing mysteries in neuropharmacology is the question as to how well do the conventional mechanisms of action for a given drug truly correlate with its biological effects, and do these mechanisms explain all pharmacological/clinical effects of a drug?

One of the most important question is as to how can drugs be used to unravel details of biochemical and physiological processes and enhance better understanding of neuropharmacology?

Lastly, what changes in the brain are responsible for bringing about relief of symptoms in Parkinson's disease, dementia, schizophrenia, depression, and multiple sclerosis and what agents are most effective in treating these conditions?

GET STARTED

There are several drug targets in neuropharmacology. The student of neuropharmacology should be able to explain or describe the pharmacodynamic principles that aid in the understanding of neural receptors and the actions of drugs on these receptors (Fig. 3.1). The second messenger systems utilized by neural receptors and how activation/inhibition of these receptors leads to a change in physiologic function (Fig. 3.2).

RECEPTORS AS DRUG TARGETS

Now, having understood the biochemical basis, let us discuss this concept in detail.

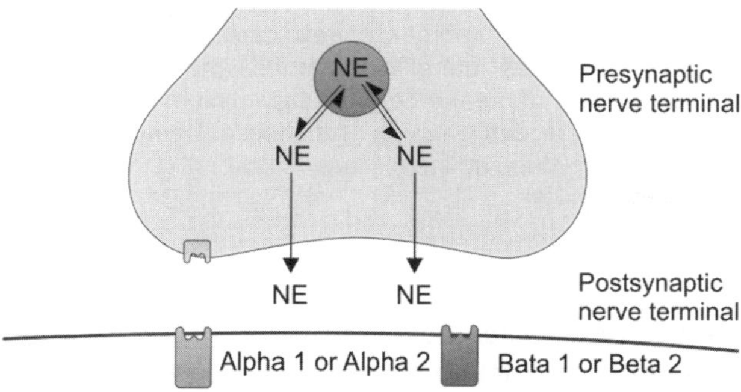

Fig. 3.1: Simplest examples of the drug targets in neuropharmacology where the drugs of autonomic nervous system act. This was the beginning hence, the drugs of this class act on a large number of receptors and produce a wide variety of pharmacological effects. (NE: norepinephrine; norepinephrine is recognized to play key role in the pathophysiology of major depressive disorder and schizophrenia)

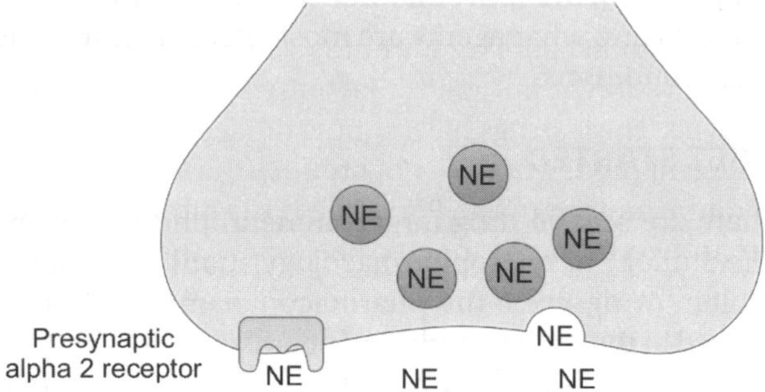

Fig. 3.2: Alpha-2 receptors, an example of adrenergic receptors present in brain are widely distributed and are target sites of drugs such as clonidine and methyldopa used in treatment of hypertension. All its subtypes (alpha-2A, alpha-2B, and alpha-2C) have locations throughout brain. These receptors are, however, not just present inside brain but throughout the body as well. Alpha-2 receptors exist presynaptically. Activation of these receptors inhibit the release of norepinephrine. The mechanism of this regulatory involves the stimulation of a G-protein gated K^+ channel leading to membrane hyperpolarization. Noradrenergic receptors are found on neurons of locus coeruleus and send their projections to forebrain, cortex, cerebellum, amygdala, hippocampus, basal ganglia, thalamus, and hypothalamus etc. Drugs can decrease (e.g. hemicholinium synthesis of acetylcholine) or can block degradation of neurotransmitter synthesis (e.g. Mono amine oxidase inhibitors).
(NE: norepinephrine)

Agonists

Agonists are drugs designed to mimic the natural messenger and act by stimulating receptors. Several drugs such as apomorphine, ropinirole are dopamine agonists.

Agonists should bind and leave quickly—number of binding interactions is important.

Partial Agonists

Partial agonists are agent binds as an agonist to one receptor subtype but as an antagonist to another receptor subtype. These drugs have submaximal efficacy.

Agent binds but does not produce the ideal induced fit for maximum effect. Partial agonists bind to binding site in two different modes, one where the agent acts as an agonist and one where it acts as an antagonist (Fig. 3.3). Examples include pentazocine, buprenorphine, bromocriptine, etc.

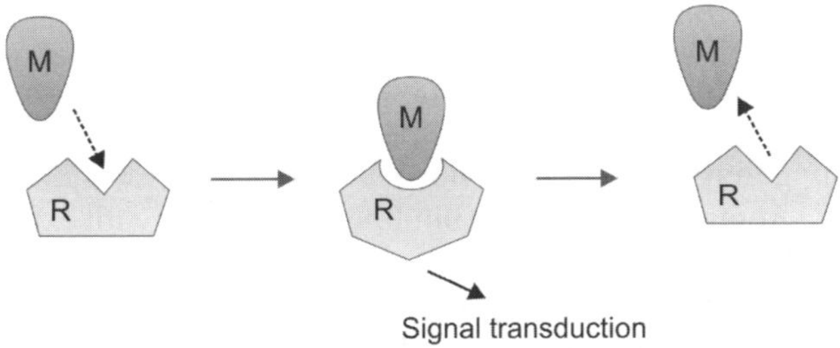

Fig. 3.3: Agonists bind reversibly to the binding site and produce the same induced fit as the natural messenger—receptor is activated. Similar intermolecular bonds formed as with natural messenger. Agonists are often similar in structure to the natural messenger. One can alter axonal conduction using local anesthetics. Similarly, alteration synaptic transmission is possible by the use of antidepressants. Many drugs affect receptors and include dopamine agonists, e.g. ropinirole. If drug causes same effect as natural process, it is termed as receptor activation. Many agonists are able to do the same. Example includes benzodiazepines that increase frequency of opening of GABAA receptors-Cl channel complex. If drug reduces or causes opposite effect to that of the naturally binding ligand then receptor deactivation can occur. Examples of the same are beta blockers used in treatment of anxiety disorders and tremors, etc.

Inverse Agonists

Bind to receptor binding sites with a different induced fit from the normal messenger. Receptor is not activated and normal messenger is blocked from binding to the binding site (Fig. 3.4). Example is beta-carboline. The drug is not an antagonist as the receptor activation is there but in opposite direction. So, it should not be confused with an antagonist.

Antagonists

Antagonists are drugs designed to block the natural messenger. Trihexyphenidyl is an antagonist of acetylcholine receptors of muscarinic type.

Antagonists tend to have stronger and/or more binding interactions, resulting in a different induced fit such that the receptor is not activated.

Antagonists can form binding interactions with extra binding regions neighboring the binding site for the natural messenger (Fig. 3.5).

Noncompetitive antagonist binds irreversibly to the binding site. Different induced fit means that the receptor is not activated. Covalent bond is formed between the

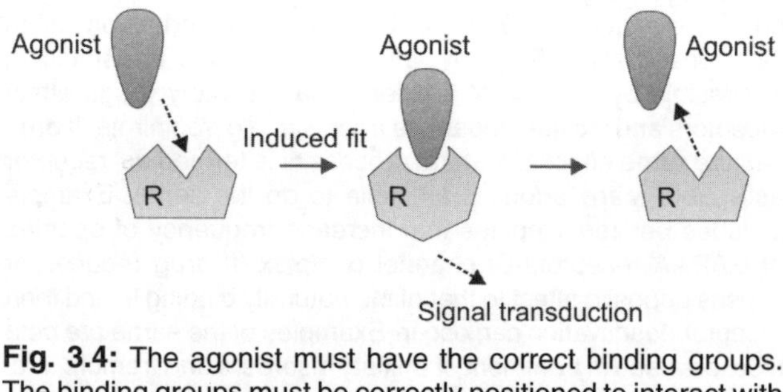

Fig. 3.4: The agonist must have the correct binding groups. The binding groups must be correctly positioned to interact with complementary binding regions. The drug must have the correct shape to fit the binding site.

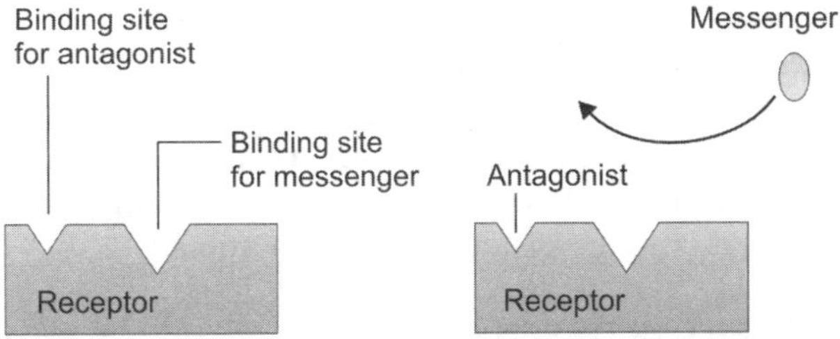

Fig. 3.5: Antagonists can form binding interactions with different receptors in vicinity to the binding site for the messenger.

drug and the receptor. Messenger is blocked from the binding site. Increasing messenger concentration does not reverse antagonism.

Competitive antagonist binds reversibly to a neighboring binding site. Intermolecular bonds formed between antagonist and binding site antagonist overlaps the messenger binding site. Messenger is blocked from the binding site.

Allosteric antagonists[1,2] bind reversibly to an allosteric binding site. Intermolecular bonds formed between antagonist and binding site induced fit alters the shape of the receptor. Binding site is distorted and is not recognized by the messenger. Increasing messenger concentration does not reverse antagonism. Allosteric modulators of G-protein coupled receptors are now being developed.[1]

RECEPTOR SENSITIZATION

Receptors may become sensitized on long-term exposure to antagonists. Cell synthesizes more receptors to compensate for blocked receptors. Cells become more sensitive to natural messenger. It can result in tolerance and dependence. Increased doses of antagonist are required to achieve same effect (tolerance). Cells are supersensitive to normal neurotransmitter and causes withdrawal symptoms when antagonist withdrawn. This leads to dependence. Receptor sensitization is now a concept undergoing extensive research in anxiety, eating disorders, post-traumatic disorders, somatoform disorders, and many neurological disorders.[3]

RECEPTOR DESENSITIZATION

Receptors become desensitized on long-term exposure to agonists. Prolonged binding of agonist leads to phosphorylation of receptor. Phosphorylated receptor changes shape and is inactivated. Dephosphorylation occurs once agonist departs. Desensitization of N-methyl-D-aspartate (NMDA) receptors by regulation of calcium release and hence modulating excitotoxicity is a potential new therapeutic target.[4] Likewise, α-amino-3-hydroxy-5-methyl-4-isoxazolepropionic acid (AMPA) receptor and gamma-aminobutyric acid (GABA) receptor desensitization strategies are being actively worked.[5,6] Adenosine receptor desensitization is another active area of potential therapeutics in neurology and psychiatry.[7]

Synaptic Transmission

Several steps are needed in synaptic transmission, a type of talk between neurons. Transmitter synthesis, transmitter storage (in the vesicles), release of transmitter (occurring in only small number of vesicles release) and the receptor binding of neurotransmitter, e.g. dopamine to its postsynaptic receptor (reversible). A given neurotransmitter once completes its action may have one of the following fates:

- Presynaptic reuptake
- Postsynaptic action (Responsible for neurotransmitter action)

- Postsynaptic reuptake
- Enzymatic degradation in synapse

Several steps are needed in synaptic transmission, a type of talk between neurons. Transmitter synthesis, transmitter storage (in the vesicles), release of transmitter (occurring in only small number of vesicles release) and the receptor binding of neurotransmitter, e.g. dopamine to its postsynaptic receptor (reversible). A given neurotransmitter once completes its action may have one of the following fates:

- Presynaptic reuptake
- Postsynaptic action (Responsible for neurotransmitter action)
- Postsynaptic reuptake
- Enzymatic degradation in synapse.

Neurotransmitters are synthesized in the presynaptic neurons and are released into synaptic cleft to stimulate or inhibit postsynaptic neurons receptors. Fast neurotransmitters (e.g. glutamate) operate through ligand-gated ion channels, slow neurotransmitters (e.g. acetylcholine-muscarinic receptors) operate through G-protein-coupled receptors.

Neuromodulators are released by neurons and supporting glial cells to produce slower pre-or postsynaptic responses (e.g. Carbon dioxide, adenosine, purines, peptides, prostaglandins, arachidonic acid and Nitric oxide).

Neuromediators are basically second messengers that play crucial role in elicitation of postsynaptic responses produced by neurotransmitters (e.g. cAMP, cGMP and inositol phosphate).

Neurotropic factors are mainly released by CNS neurons, and microglia and act longer than neuromodulators to regulate the growth and morphology of neurons and control long-term changes in brain mainly by affecting gene transcription by acting through tyrosine kinase-linked receptors (e.g. Cytokines, chemokines, growth factors).

CONCLUSION

New therapeutic targets in clinical neurology are being actively searched. For example, in Parkinson's disease adenosine receptor antagonists are being developed for quite sometime now.[8] Similarly, tumor necrosis factor (TNF)-alpha blockers are being developed for treatment of sciatica now.[9]

REFERENCES

1. Conn PJ, Christopoulos A, Lindsley CW. Allosteric modulators of GPCRs: a novel approach for the treatment of CNS disorders. Nat Rev Drug Discov. 2009;8(1):41-54.
2. Wenthur CJ, Gentry PR, Mathews TP, et al. Drugs for allosteric sites on receptors. Annu Rev Pharmacol Toxicol. 2014;54:165-84.
3. D'Alessandro G, Cerritelli F, Cortelli P. Sensitization and interoception as key neurological concepts in osteopathy and other manual medicines. Front Neurosci. 2016;10:100.
4. Sornarajah L, Vasuta OC, Zhang L, et al. NMDA receptor desensitization regulated by direct binding to PDZ1-2 domains of PSD-95. J Neurophysiol. 2008;99(6):3052-62.
5. Bianchi MT, Macdonald RL. Slow phases of GABAA receptor desensitization: structural determinants and possible relevance for synaptic function. J Physiol. 2002;544(Pt 1):3-18.
6. AMPA receptor desensitization. (2017). [online] Available from https://books.google.co.in/books?id=czzuBwAAQBAJ&pg=PA53&lpg=PA53&dq=receptor+desensitization+neurology&source=bl&ots=w1tq9yw6P5&sig=_gyrI68Dmg4Uoknvu3LL_uPyiZw&hl=en&sa=X&ved=0ahUKEwiwpZvD48bVAhUDpo8KHQaJCUcQ6AEISDAE#v=onepage&q=receptor%20desensitization%20neurology&f=false. [Accessed May, 2018].

7. Adenosine receptor desensitization. (2017). [online] Available from https://books.google.co.in/books?id=pgZ0AwAAQBAJ&pg=PA331&lpg=PA331&dq=receptor+desensitization+neurology&source=bl&ots=T452RVob-Y&sig=Y0mbTQe0vdYLpCInSq0m0QRfgVo&hl=en&sa=X&ved=0ahUKEwiwpZvD48bVAhUDpo8KHQaJCUcQ6AEIQDAC#v=onepage&q= receptor%20desensitization%20neurology&f = false. [Accessed May, 2018].
8. Armentero MT, Pinna A, Ferré S, et al. Past, present and future of A(2A) adenosine receptor antagonists in the therapy of Parkinson's disease. Pharmacol Ther. 2011;132(3):280-99.
9. Wang YF, Chen PY, Chang W, et al. Clinical significance of tumor necrosis factor-α inhibitors in the treatment of sciatica: a systematic review and meta-analysis. PLoS One. 2014;9(7):e103147.

CHAPTER

4

Clinical Pharmacokinetics

INTRODUCTION

Pharmacokinetics means movement of drugs in the body. Drugs once given by any systemic routes will reach the bloodstream if the systemic effect is desired. Pharmacokinetics has four components: (1) absorption, (2) distribution, (3) metabolism, and (4) elimination (ADME). All of them have considerable importance in clinical neurology.

ABSORPTION

Entry into circulation is absorption. For oral route, the drug has to pass various barriers like stomach and intestine. For drugs given intravenously, the drug goes to circulation directly.

Most common mode of drug absorption of the drugs given by oral route (which is most common) is *passive diffusion.* It depends upon lipid solubility. Water-soluble drugs are absorbed across pores in cell membranes of intestines. Absorption of many antiepileptic drugs may be reduced by calcium containing antacids.

Active transport depends upon expense of adenosine triphosphate (ATP) hence is saturable. Drugs like levodopa are absorbed via this method.

Facilitated absorption is also known as cotransport and is seen in case of drugs like 5-fluorouracil used in treatment of cancers.

Most of the drugs are absorbed from upper part of small intestine. Some drugs can get absorbed from stomach as well. Drugs like aspirin, used in stroke prevention can get absorbed via stomach. These drugs may have acidic nature. An acidic drug, at acidic pH will remain nonionized as per Henderson-Hasselbalch equation. Therefore, absorption can be good.

Absorption of drugs like diazepam occurs via rectal mucosal membrane.

Bioavailability is amount of drug going in circulation without metabolism. It depends upon many factors. Since there can be brand to brand variations in bioavailability; therefore, in case of drugs like phenytoin, carbamazepine, and lithium one should always use same brand. Brand to brand variation in drugs like phenytoin can even cause drug failure and breakthrough seizures.

DISTRIBUTION

It means spread of the drug. Once a drug enters into blood, it goes to various places in the body. However, some drugs go to a perfused organ such as brain and then come to plasma again. This is known as *redistribution.* An anesthetic agent thiopentone undergoes quick redistribution hence is a short-acting drug. *Redistribution* makes drugs short acting as the drug quickly leaves the organ it intends to work upon. Hence, it indicates metabolism of drug.

Distribution can be quantified by knowing about volume of distribution (Vd).

Vd = Dose of drug/concentration

i.e. it depends upon dose given and concentration achieved in blood. Drugs can have low Vd (<5 liters) or high Vd (>5 liters). Drugs with high Vd cannot be removed by hemodialysis in case of poisoning as the drug has high Vd and it is outside blood and is there is tissues. That is why, dialysis is not useful in digoxin overdose (Vd = 420 liters).

Tissue Storage

Some tissues like eye, receive good amount of certain drugs like amiodarone that gets deposited in cornea. Similarly, drugs like chloroquine get deposited in retina leading to interference with color vision (Bull's eye maculopathy).

Protein Binding

All drugs that are able to enter into bloodstream are bound to plasma proteins which represent temporary storage of drugs. Acidic drugs are bound to albumin and basic to alpha-1 glycoproteins. Protein bound drugs are neither metabolized nor eliminated. Drug displacement can occur here. A drug that has high affinity can displace a drug with lower affinity of protein binding. Like aspirin binds tightly to protein albumin and can displace methotrexate from protein binding. Likewise, if sodium valproate is given to patients taking phenytoin then displacement can occur.

Barriers

All the drugs that enter into bloodstream will try to enter into various tissues or organs. Blood-brain barrier is the toughest barrier, while blood-placenta barrier is weakest barrier. Drugs like atropine, insulin, and heparin, however, do not enter blood-placenta barrier hence are safe in pregnancy.

METABOLISM

It means inactivation of drugs. However, some drugs are activated in body and are known as *prodrugs*.

Example of *prodrugs:*

- Levodopa → Methyldopa
- Prednisone → Prednisolone
- Enalapril → Enalaprilat
- Hydroxyzine → Cetirizine
- Terfenadine → Cetirizine
- Oxcarbazepine → Carbamazepine.

Active drugs are able to exert pharmacological effects.

Drugs like carbamazepine, oxcarbazepine may form active metabolites. Drugs like gabapentin, however, do not undergo any metabolism and are eliminated unchanged by kidneys (Fig. 4.1).[1]

Metabolism or bioinactivation is a phasic process and involves two different phases: (1) phase I and (2) phase II.

Phase I involves changing functional character of drug and phase II involves conjugating the drug with an endogenous compound (e.g. glycine, acetic acid, glutathione, etc.). Nature has ensured that there is a strong covalent bond between drug and the endogenous compound so that the drug is finally eliminated from the body. Ultimate aim of metabolism is to convert a lipid-soluble drug into a water-soluble drug. It is important to know that large fluctuations in concentrations of some drugs like antiepileptic drugs in children and elderly are possible.

Drugs are metabolized by liver enzymes known as cytochromal enzymes and have more than 60 isoforms and 14 families. Some drugs like atracurium

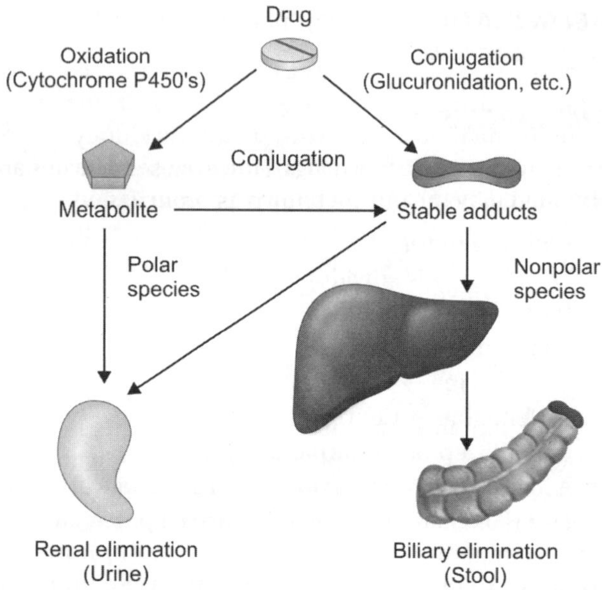

Fig. 4.1: A drug is exposed to liver enzymes and is broken down to inactive or active products (sometimes). Finally products can be eliminated via urine or kidneys.

are metabolized without enzymes and are known as Hoffman's elimination.

Some drugs like rifampin can act as enzyme inducers and can increase metabolism of concomitantly administered drugs. Other drugs like ketoconazole act as enzyme inhibitors and increase plasma levels of other drugs. This approach can be clinically used. For example, ritonavir is used to treat human immunodeficiency virus (HIV) infection. It has the ability of inhibiting metabolism of other drugs. It is given along with other drugs and can increase plasma levels of other drugs and this can be useful in using lower than usual dose of other drugs without causing significant toxicity.

ELIMINATION

It means removal of drugs. Kidneys are most common organs of drug removal. *Glomerular filtration* is most common method of drug elimination via kidneys. Some drugs like penicillin (acidic) and digoxin (basic) are eliminated by tubular secretion in proximal convoluted tubules. Some drugs that are highly lipid soluble are reabsorbed and become long-acting. Hence, kidneys are thoroughly involved in drug elimination.

Some drugs that are short acting like penicillins become long-acting if these are given with probenecid. It is noteworthy that probenecid can inhibit elimination of penicillin and make it longer acting. This is useful clinically. However, quinidine can interfere with renal elimination of penicillin and thus can lead to toxicity. Dose of digoxin may, therefore, have to be reduced.

Clearance

It means making plasma free from drug per unit time. It is an important pharmacokinetic concept.

CL = Rate of elimination/plasma concentration

As the drugs are removed by a liver, kidneys, and some other organs like lungs; therefore, clearance of drugs is additive by nature. Drugs are mainly eliminated by two different manners: (1) zero order and (2) first order.

Zero order is fixed amount eliminated per unit time. Drugs eliminated by this method are handled by enzymes that have saturable nature. Therefore, the drugs if given in high dose can lead to toxicity. Drugs of this nature are slowly increased in dose. Monitoring of plasma levels is required. Some drugs follow zero order in high dose and is known as pseudozero order. Examples include aspirin, theophylline, and phenytoin.

First order is most common method of drug elimination. It means a constant fraction of plasma is made free from the drug per unit time. Both clearance and half-life in this form of drug elimination remains fixed while they change in zero order.

HALF-LIFE

It means plasma concentration of a drug dips by half in a given time. A drug leaves the body in 4–5 half-lives until it is repeated. About 90% of drug leaves the body in 3–4 half-lives. It is a good estimator of interdose interval.
It is calculated by:

$t/1/2 = 0.693 \times Vd/Cl$

Where Vd is volume of distribution, Cl is clearance.
0.693 is elimination constant.

Half-life is an important pharmacokinetic parameters and helps us in knowing:

- Duration of drug action.
- Interdose interval (how frequently do we need to give the drug).
- Time in which a drug achieves steady state in blood.

However, it does not tell us anything about drug dose.
Dosages can be calculated by following formulas:

- *Loading dose*: Calculated by:
  Vd × desired concentrations.
- *Maintenance dose*:
  Cl × concentrations.

Loading dose is not affected in renal failure, while maintenance dose is reduced in renal failure as clearance is reduced in renal failure.

SPECIAL ISSUES IN PHARMACOKINETICS IN NEUROLOGY[2,3]

Drugs like phenytoin have narrow therapeutic index, hence their drug monitoring is needed. Phenytoin is

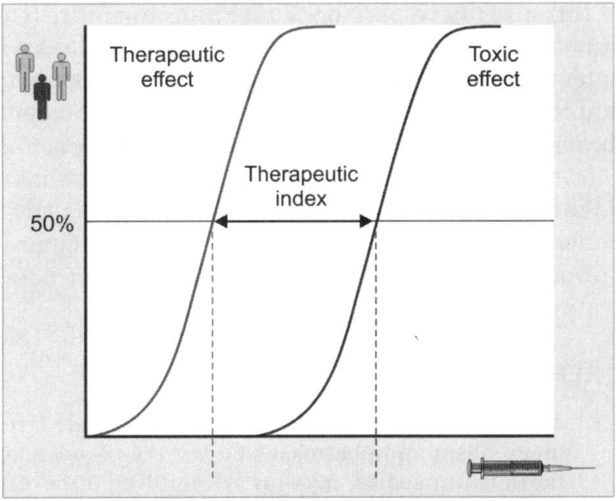

Fig. 4.2: Therapeutic index is a therapeutic ratio and is actually a ratio between therapeutic to toxicity ratio.

highly protein bound and only unbound drug is able to enter blood-brain barrier, hence some correction of dosing is needed in patients with hypoalbuminemia. This can maximize efficacy but minimizes toxicity. Detailed calculations can be found here.[4]

Therapeutic Index[5]

It is ratio between lethal dose in 50% of animals to drug dose producing 50% of maximal effect in humans (LD50/ED50). Drugs having narrow therapeutic index will require monitoring (Fig. 4.2). Many neurological drugs like phenytoin, lithium have a narrow therapeutic index.

CONCLUSION

Drugs used in the treatment of central nervous system, diseases have a unique ability to enter in the brain (e.g. Antideprssants, antipsychotic, etc). Some of the drugs of this class have very poor oral bioavailability (e.g. Levodopa) due to intestinal metabolism. Some drugs enter the brain but come out quickly, e.g. Thiopentone, flumazenil (redistribution). This can lead to shortening of duration of action. Drugs like fluoxetine are long acting, allowing once daily or even once weekly administration. Volume of distribution of this class of drugs is large, hence hemodialysis may not be a good therapeutic option in overdose and patients have to be treated symptomatically.

REFERENCES

1. Alavijeh MS, Chishty M, Qaiser MZ, et al. Drug metabolism and pharmacokinetics, the blood-brain barrier, and central nervous system drug discovery. NeuroRx. 2005;2(4):554-71.
2. Browne TR. Pharmacokinetics of antiepileptic drugs. Neurology. 1998;51(5 Suppl 4):S2-7.
3. Edward FJ. (2017). Pharmacodynamic and pharmacokinetic principles of pharmacology and drug therapy. [online] Available from http://journals.lww.com/jnpt/Abstract/2003/27030/Pharmacodynamic_and_Pharmacokinetic_Principles_of.3.aspx. [Accessed May, 2018].
4. ClinCalc. (2017). Phenytoin correction calculator. [online] Available from http://clincalc.com/Phenytoin/Correction.aspx. [Accessed May, 2018].
5. Tamargo J, Le Heuzey JY, Mabo P. Narrow therapeutic index drugs: a clinical pharmacological consideration to flecainide. Eur J Clin Pharmacol. 2015;71(5):549-67.

CHAPTER

5

Clinical Pharmacodynamics

HISTORY OF DRUG ACTION IN CENTRAL NERVOUS SYSTEM

Drugs acting on nerves are among the first few drugs discovered by humans. These drugs not only have been aimed at easing illness but also have been developed for improving sense of well-being. Approximately one-fourth of all drugs used around the world have their site of action at central nervous system.[1-4]

MECHANISMS

The mechanisms by which neurological drugs work are not always clear. However, in recent times, good deal of understanding has emerged due to which the probability of developing further drugs has increased. Given here is the summary of drug action mechanisms needed for understanding the same.

Pharmacodynamics means mechanism of action of drugs. Drug action in clinical neurology is very important for proper understanding of pharmacotherapy of neurological disorders.

SYNAPSES AS THE MAIN SITE OF ACTION IN NEUROLOGY

There are various sites of drug action but the synapses are the main site of action in neurology.

Drugs acting in central nervous system could be summarized to act upon:

- Presynaptic
- Postsynaptic.

Presynaptic strategies involve altering the levels of neurotransmitter in the synaptic cleft. This can be achieved by changing the amount of endogenous neurotransmitter released or available for release into the synaptic cleft, or by altering the amount of neurotransmitter taken back up (reuptake) into the presynaptic terminal. This is best achieved by drugs like selective serotonin reuptake inhibitors (SSRIs). SSRIs are extensively used in psychiatry.

In neurology, the dopaminergic synapse can be used as a specific example to illustrate mechanism of action.

- *Blockade of dopamine metabolism:* For example, monoamine oxidase B inhibitors, such as selegiline or rasagiline, block dopamine degradation, hence making more dopamine available for release.
- *Inhibition of dopamine synthesis:* Inhibitors of dopamine synthesis, such as α-methyltyrosine, reduce the amount of dopamine available for release. Drugs like reserpine and tetrabenazine decrease vesicular-mediated release by blocking vesicular monoamine transporters, which prevents the storage of neurotransmitter into synaptic vesicles.
- *Dopamine transporter block:* Inhibitors of membrane dopamine transporters, such as bupropion or

cocaine, block the reuptake of dopamine from the synapse, and thereby, keep levels of dopamine in the synaptic cleft high.

- *Psychostimulants:* Certain drugs, which are extensively used as psychostimulant, e.g. amphetamine, cause dopamine release by running the DA transporter in reverse.
- *Autoreceptors:* In some cases, receptors are located on presynaptic terminals that bind the neurotransmitter being released, e.g. a dopamine receptor located on a presynaptic dopaminergic terminal. When these so-called autoreceptors are stimulated they reduce the release of neurotransmitters, and when blocked they increase neurotransmitter release.

Postsynaptic actions: In contrast to presynaptic strategies, which alter the levels of endogenous neurotransmitter in the synaptic cleft, postsynaptic strategies modulate neurotransmission with chemical agents that act directly on postsynaptic receptors.

Drugs could:
- Stimulate (amphetamines stimulate brain)
- Depress (benzodiazepines depress brain).

To achieve this, drugs act via various mechanisms:
- *Agonist*: Drugs stimulating receptors are known as agonists. These have intrinsic activity (efficacy) and affinity (binding ability).
  - *Full agonists*: Drugs like adrenalin have intrinsic activity and thus are able to activate heart. Hence, a subcutaneous injection of adrenalin is used in anaphylactic shock. Dopamine agonists are used for Parkinson's disease and restless legs syndrome.
  - *Partial agonists*: Some drugs may have dual activity (agonist-antagonist) such as tamoxifen and can block estrogenic receptors on breast and

stimulate same receptors on bones and uterus. Drugs like sumatriptan, etc. are examples.
  - *Inverse agonists*: These drugs are drugs having intrinsic activity in opposite direction. Beta-carbolines are one such example.
- *Antagonist*:
  - *Reversible*: This form of antagonism is known as surmountable. That means, like effect of acetylcholine can be reversed by using atropine which is a competitive antagonist of acetylcholine. High dose of either of them can block effect of each other.
  - *Irreversible*: This is a strong form of antagonism in which the drug binds to its receptors tightly and is virtually inseparable. Example of this form of antagonism includes phenoxybenzamine which is used for a rare tumor pheochromocytoma.

To achieve various pharmacological effects, drugs could act via several receptors:
- *Receptors*: Basically, these are protein molecules but almost any component of the cells machinery could act as receptors nowadays.
  - *G-protein coupled receptors*: These are most common receptors. Drugs could activate stimulatory (Gs) or inhibitory G proteins (Gs) or quite type (Gq). Depending upon the nature of action, the drugs could increase formation of either of the following:
    - Cyclic adenosine monophosphate (cAMP)
    - Cyclic guanosine monophosphate (cGMP)
    - Inositol 1,4,5-trisphosphate (IP3)/Diacylglycerol (DAG).

  Chemicals mentioned earlier that are generated in response to drugs are known as *secondary messengers*. These mediate pharmacological effects of a variety of drugs. Types of receptors are given in Box 5.1.

Box 5.1: Types of receptors.

- Voltage-gated channels
- Ligand-gated channels
- Ionotropic receptors
- Metabotropic receptors.

- *Ionotropic receptors*: There is no secondary messenger involved here. Drugs could open or close receptors that act as ion channels here.
- *Cytokine receptors*: As the name suggests, receptors could move inside the cell membranes. These are coupled to special secondary messengers like Janus kinase-Signal transducers and activators of transcription (JAK-STAT) pathways. Drugs like erythropoietin stimulate them.
- *Growth factor receptors*: Insulin is most important drug acting via these receptors. Drug binds to alpha subunits extracellularly, and drugs could produce pharmacological effects intracellularly phosphorylating beta subunits. This can initiate changes in intracellular enzymes, etc.
- *Intranuclear receptors*: Drugs, steroids and sex hormones, vitamins (vitamin A and D), and thyroid hormones (T3/T4) act via these receptors. Drug binds intracellularly to cytoplasmic receptors. Drug and receptor complex then migrates to nucleus and finally change gene expression. Since these drugs are acting via change in gene expression, therefore, there is a latency of clinical response and do not act immediately.

SYNERGISTIC DRUG ACTION

Drugs could act if these are given together. Sometimes, it may not be possible to use high dose of a drug due to side effects in this case, two drugs can be combined so that side effects do not add up but pharmacological effects could get added up.

It is of two types:

1. *Addition*: Two drugs are used, and their effects add up but side effects do not add. A popular combination is ibuprofen and paracetamol (e.g. *combiflam*) has two drugs with two different mechanisms/purposes. Ibuprofen is anti-inflammatory and paracetamol is a good analgesic. Combination of both of them provides good analgesia with anti-inflammatory effect.
2. *Potentiation*: It means one drug is inactive and other drug is active. Examples include levodopa and carbidopa. Levodopa is active, while carbidopa just inhibits extracerebral metabolism of levodopa. Thus, levodopa becomes a long-acting drug.

DOSE-RESPONSE CURVE

Mathematical relationship between long of dose and response produced is known as *dose-response curve* (DRC). Normal shape of DRC is sigmoid (Fig. 5.1).

Dose-response curve is a tool to evaluate safety, efficacy, and tolerability of drugs in a clinical setup. DRC for therapeutic effects may be different from side effects. X-axis gives an idea about potency. Shift to left means more potent and shift to right means less. Parallel and right shift is done by competitive antagonists. Flat DRC is seen in case of irreversible antagonists. Slope of DRC tells us about safety of drugs. Steep DRC means unsafe drugs and flat DRC means safe drugs.

FACTORS AFFECTING DRUG ACTION

- *Age*: Pharmacological effects may be exaggerated in young infants as the pathways for metabolism or

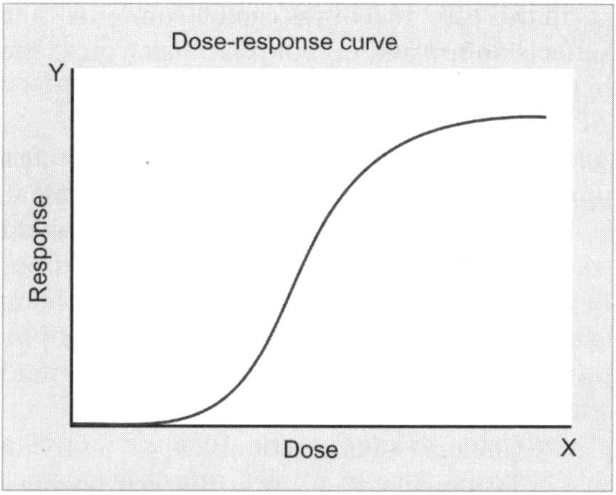

Fig. 5.1: Dose-response curve (DRC). Normally it is sigmoid. X-axis indicates dose and Y-axis indicates response. Slope of DRC indicates safety of drug.

elimination may not be properly developed. Moreover, in elderly, drugs responses may be higher as pathways that were once established now degenerate.

- *Genetics*: Certain enzymes that metabolize the drugs may not be present in individuals or may be present but defective. This may lead to aberration in handling the drug. For example, glucose-6-phosphate dehydrogenase (G6PD), an enzyme that maintains the integrity of red blood cell (RBC) membranes that can lead to hemolytic crises. Drugs like benzhexol and levodopa have been linked with hemolytic crises in G6PD apart from antimalarials which are common causes of hemolysis in this genetic condition.
- *Pregnancy*: Some drugs are bad during pregnancy and can cause defective formation of organs. These are known as teratogenic. Examples include:
  - *Bad (teratogenic drugs) in pregnancy*:
    - Thalidomide → Phocomelia
    - Valproate → Neural tube defects

  - Lithium → Ebstein's abnormality (abnormal heart valves)
  - Phenytoin → Cleft palate, lip, and microcephaly
  - Corticosteroids → Cardiac defects
  - Levodopa → Visceral and skeletal abnormalities
  - Enalapril → Fetopathy (renal agenesis)
  - Propranolol → Intrauterine growth retardation.
- *Therapeutic drugs in pregnancy*:
  - Fever → Paracetamol
  - Pain → Diclofenac
  - Amebiasis
  - Giardiasis
  - Cholera → Furazolidone
  - Typhoid fever → Ampicillin/ceftriaxone
  - Malaria → Chloroquine
  - Epilepsy → Phenobarbitone
  - Hypertension → Methyldopa.

DRUG DISCOVERY AND DEVELOPMENT

This is a tedious process and taken almost 1 billion US dollars to develop a single drug. That is why, in countries like India not many drugs are developed.

To develop a drug, a lead molecule is found based upon screening of a large number of compounds. Once a promising compound is found, then it is subjected to animal testing. Lot of tests like acute and chronic toxicity studies are done. Medicines are fed to pregnant animals and teratogenicity is noted. Once a drug is cleared, then it enters *clinical trials*.

Clinical trials are human experiments involving a minimum of 20 subjects.

- *Phase I*: Pharmacokinetics and safety of drug evaluated.
- *Phase II*: Safety + pharmacokinetic evaluated. Nowadays, it is used for efficacy testing as well.

- *Phase III*: Efficacy tested.
- *Phase IV*: Postmarketing surveillance done.

INDIAN PHARMACOPOEIA

This is an official publication regarding medicines of Ministry of Health and Family Welfare, Government of India. It regularly updates the existing information about medicines used in India. It also sets standards for drugs usage. It also promotes use of generic medications by publishing national formulary. Abbreviation IP denotes Indian Pharmacopoeia like British Pharmacopoeia (BP) and United States Pharmacopeia (USP) or British National Formulary (BNF). This was first published in the year 1955 and in 2010, its 6th edition was published.

Legal Issues

Indian Pharmacopoeia is a legal body, having a governing body, general body, and a scientific body as well.

Drugs and Cosmetic Act, 1940

This contains 168 rules and schedule from A to Y. Most important schedule is schedule H which includes prescription drugs. A doctor's prescription is needed for obtaining schedule H drugs. Likewise, schedule E includes poisonous substances to be used under different systems of alternative medicines in India. It mainly deals and regulates:

- Adulterations in medicines
- Misbranding
- Spurious drugs
- Standards of quality
- Disclosure of name/s of manufacturer
- Provisions related to alternative system of medicine.

RATIONAL DRUGS USE IN NEUROLOGY

Safe and reliable administration of medicines is the responsibility of nurses once drugs are prescribed. Though drugs are prescribed traditionally by doctors, in some countries such as England limited prescription is allowed for nurses. In India, doctors prescribe and nurses play a vital role in administering medicines to patients. Medicines in hospitals are usually kept in custody and they dispense or release in wards. In some hospital, this role may be taken up by pharmacists.

Following are nurses role in managing drug uses in hospital or outpatient departments (OPDs):

- *Storing medicines in wards/outpatient departments*: Generally there are warehouses in hospital units where drugs are stored and kept in recommended conditions. It may be useful to read prescribing information for drugs that residents are not very familiar with before administering.
- *Dispensing to general staff*: Drugs are released by ward incharge upon demands to all the nurses working in a hospital ward. This depends upon the patient load and particular prescription. These could be stored in the local fridge or cupboard for immediate use. Medicines are indented and this letter is sent to hospital pharmacist who intern will supply medicines to hospital ward.
- *Reading and recording prescription*: Prescriptions are written by physicians on OPD cards and on hospital ward sheet. These are kept together and tagged near bedside for ready reference. Further orders are written on these sheets and are used to administer drugs to patients.
- *Administering medicines*: This is the most important responsibility of nurses in hospitals, wards, and in clinical units. Proper care must be taken to ensure

that instructions of doctors are read properly and clarified in case of doubts. In the earlier chapter on routes of drug administration, details are given about various methods via which medicines can be given. Figure 5.2 gives introduction to drugs administration.

- *Taking proper drug history*: A proper history taking is vitally important and this ensures that history of drug allergy is recorded. In future, therefore, such drugs are avoided to that patient.
- *Teaching patients about drugs and their side effects*: Teaching patients, their relatives about the correct method of drug administration, giving advices about monitoring of drug therapy, and reporting

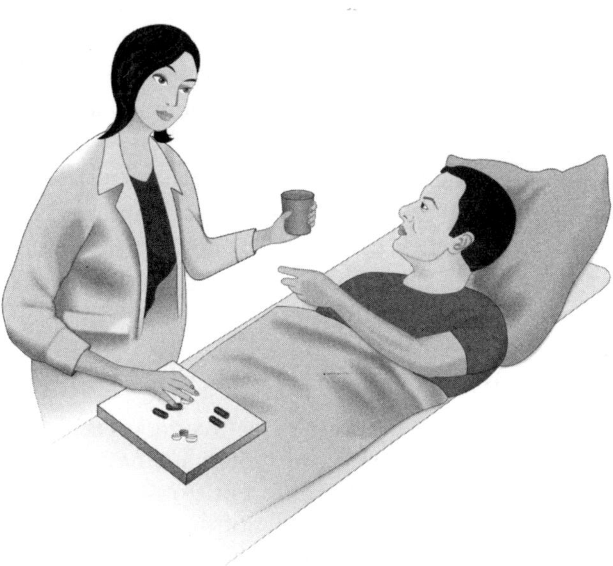

Fig. 5.2: Administering medicines properly, timely and teaching patients about correct method of taking medicines, and about their side effects are major responsibilities of nurses in Indian hospitals.

when some side effects occur are some of the main responsibilities of nurses.

Administering medicines properly like *right dose, right patient, and right time* is critically important. Following may be a useful scheme that could be followed in hospital setting. Though these are general rules, but they are as applicable to neurology like any other branch as well.[4] The given here suggestions may seem elementary but they work well:

- Read patient's full name
- Read prescription thoroughly
- Check label of drug, see expiry date
- Read proper dose and measure correct amount to be taken
- Recheck label before returning
- Do not mix two drugs in same syringe
- Two nurses can identify patient's identity in case of doubt
- Ensure patient is in fit state to receive the drug
- Periodically check patients vitals and infusion rate in case patient is getting intravenous (IV) infusion
- Record the date, time, and sign after you have administered the drug.

CONCLUSION

Drugs acting in the brain act on wide variety of receptors. The ability to affect neurotransmitter synthesis, storage and release makes them different from other drugs. Additionally, many if not most of them produce side effects that may need monitoring. Moreover, dosages used in Indian patients may be different from the western population. Moreover, these are given for a long time. Hence, understanding pharmacological basis of their drug is essential to better prescription.

REFERENCES

1. Gray JA, Nicoll RA (2017). Introduction to the pharmacology of CNS drugs. [online] Available from https://accessmedicine.mhmedical.com/Content.aspx?bookId=1193&sectionId=69106670. [Accessed May, 2018].
2. von Graevenitz KS, Shulman LM, Revell SP. Levodopa in pregnancy. Mov Disord. 1996;11(1):115-6.
3. Schetz JA. Pharmacotherapeutic principles of neurological and psychiatric disorders. In: Tarazi FI, Schetz JA (Eds). Current Clinical Neurology: Neurological and Psychiatric Disorders: From Bench to Bedside. New Jersey: Humana Press Inc.; 2005.
4. World Health Organization (WHO). (2006). Neurological disorders: Public health challenges. [online] Available from www.who.int/mental_health/neurology/neurological_disorders_report_web.pdf. [Accessed May, 2018].

CHAPTER

6

Drug Treatment of Headaches

INTRODUCTION

Headache affects up to 25% and grades of severity may vary from mild to severe. Some patients have daily or near-daily headache making the prevalence as 90% or more. Tension headache is by far the most common cause of headache. Almost half of adults had a headache in last year or so. Headaches thus account for significant morbidity and lost productivity,[1] even though they remain undiagnosed and untreated as per estimates of World Health Organization.

Limited physician training, limited access to care, inappropriate or incomplete treatment and underestimation of headache morbidity are some of the common reasons of failures of headache treatments.

PRINCIPLES OF HEADACHE TREATMENT

One would have start by ruling out potentially dangerous (secondary) headache. Serious causes include neoplasm, infection, hemorrhage, etc. One would have to take thorough history and physical examination. Three cornerstone of headache treatment are: (1) diagnose headache types, (2) implement treatments, and (3) monitor outcomes.[2]

SECONDARY HEADACHES

These are not common headaches and account for less than 2% of headaches in primary care offices. Causes are given in Box 6.1 while Box 6.2 gives list of warning causes of headaches.[3-5]

PRIMARY HEADACHES

Primary headaches usually involve an intrinsic dysfunction of the nervous system. Most patients presenting to primary care doctors with headache have

Box 6.1: Causes of secondary headaches.[3]

- Head trauma
- Vascular disease
- Neoplasms
- Substance abuse or withdrawal
- Infection/inflammation
- Metabolic disorders.

Box 6.2: Warning signs in headaches.[4,5]

- First or worst headache (*thunderclap headache*)
- Progressive or new daily persistent headache
- Age more than 50 years or less than 5 years
- Headache associated with fever, rash, and stiff neck
- Headache associated with abnormal mental status or abnormal neurological examination
- Headache associated with papilledema
- New onset headache in patient with malignancy, immunosuppression/human immunodeficiency virus (HIV), or pregnancy
- Sleep interruption due to headache
- Headache with Valsalva or exertion.

primary headache syndromes. Episodic headache is, however, more common. Chronic headache is defined as attacks occurring more frequently than 15 days/month for more than 6 months.

DIAGNOSIS OF HEADACHE

First things first, one would have to rule out secondary headache. This is done using thorough history, neurological, and musculoskeletal examinations. Imaging, blood investigations, and/or cerebrospinal analysis are done if "red flag(s)" (warning signs-see earlier) are found.

DIAGNOSE HEADACHE TYPE

One can begin by identifying comorbid illnesses, area of head involved, pain quality, and severity. Other symptoms (nausea, vomiting, and light sensitivity) and triggers may give clue to the cause of headache, e.g. tension headache or migraine. One should always pay attention to the timing (including perimenstrual). Preheadache warning symptoms (*aura*)—for example, visual changes, etc. could indicate migraine, details of which are given here.

Migraine

Migraine is a *neurological disorder* in which, the brain becomes hypersensitive and overly responsive to stimuli. The *trigeminal nerve* appears to be a key pathway activated. Vasoactive substances inflame vascular and meningeal tissues, activate trigeminal axons leading to vasodilation and headache.

Pathophysiology

Perivascular release of vasoactive neuropeptides, spreading neurogenic inflammation appears to dilate blood vessels (Fig. 6.1).

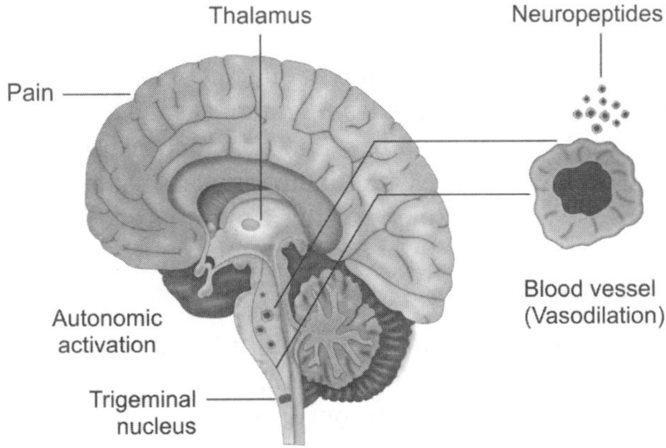

Fig. 6.1: Pathophysiology of migraine involves activation of trigeminovascular mechanisms leading to vasodilation and headache. The inflammatory response spreads along the trigeminovascular system and pain signals reach trigeminal nucleus caudalis and other pain systems. Dorsal raphe nucleus may modulate migraine pain.

Clinical Features

Migraine[5] is episodic, progressive head pain which is pulsating, throbbing, and stabbing. The attacks may last for up to 72 hours. Migraine is unilateral in about two-thirds of cases and up to 75% may have neck pain.

Migraine has female preponderance (3:1 female:male ratio) and family history is found in majority of cases. Onset of migraine occurs typically during adolescence or young adulthood. Onset after age 40 years is possible but is not common (may be relieved by menopause). Common triggers include hormonal fluctuations and hence perimenstrual migraine is very common. Weather changes, diet, including missed meals, and stress are common factors leading to precipitation of migraine attacks.

Migraine Types

Migraine with aura is found in one out of five cases and neurologic event precedes migraine (usually by 30–60 minutes). Visual, auditory, and olfactory disturbances may occur. Migraine without aura is seen in majority of cases. No aura or other warning symptoms occur.

Chronic Migraine

Chronic migraine starts as episodic migraine and attacks occur at increasing frequency. Eventually a dozen or more attacks/month can occur. Frequent association with *medication overuse* can occur and psychiatric comorbidity is common.

Management of Migraine[6,7]

Principles of migraine treatment: The management starts by educating the migraine patients and the use of migraine-specific agents in moderate to severe disease. One should use nonoral route for patients with significant nausea and vomiting. Also, one has to be aware of medication overuse and rebound in case the patient has been using over the counter drugs in long run.

When to treat?

This is an important question and the answer is simple, i.e. as early as possible. The general accepted window is within 2 hours. Treatment during prodrome or aura is even more effective.

Nonsteroidal anti-inflammatory drugs (NSAIDs) are usually the drugs of first choice in migraine treatment (Box 6.3). The National Institute of Clinical Excellence (NICE), UK recommends triptans with or without NSAIDs in acute attack of migraine. Ergots are no

Box 6.3: Commonly used nonsteroidal anti-inflammatory drugs (NSAIDs) in acute migraine.

- Ibuprofen
- Naproxen
- Diclofenac
- Tolfenamic acid
- Indomethacin
- Aspirin
- Combinations of NSAIDs (e.g. naproxen + domperidone).

TABLE 6.1: Doses of acute antimigraine drugs.

Sumatriptan	50–100 mg oral
Zolmitriptan	2.5 mg oral
Aspirin	1,000 mg oral
Ibuprofen	400 mg oral
Naproxen	500 mg oral
Paracetamol	500/650 mg oral

longer recommended in acute treatment of migraine. Metoclopramide or prochlorperazine are recommended for those patients who are either vomiting or are unable to tolerate oral therapy. Subcutaneous or nasal triptans are recommended for those who fail on initial drugs.

Nonsteroidal anti-inflammatory drugs: If severe symptoms present then one should not try over the counter drugs. Research work has shown improved outcomes with migraine-specific therapy in such cases. One can consider route of administration and also consider contraindications while prescribing these drugs, e.g. avoiding ergot alkaloids in patients with ischemic heart disease. Dosages of antimigraine drugs used in acute migraine are given in Table 6.1.

Flowchart 6.1: Management of migraine. Note that NSAIDS are the mainstay of mild to moderate cases and triptans/other drugs are used in severe cases.

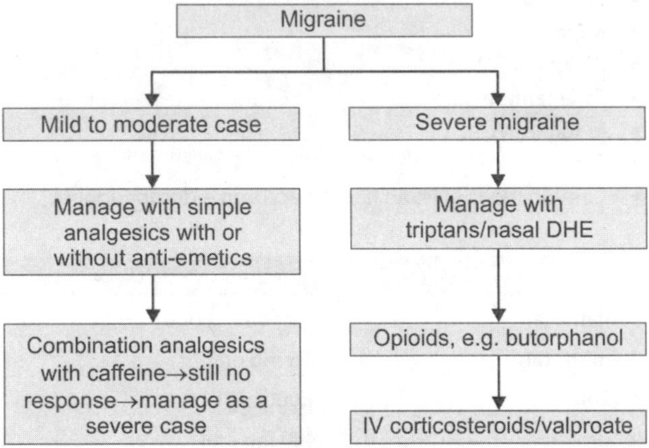

Triptans: After NSAIDs, these have become preferred drugs (Flowchart 6.1). These are more effective than NSAIDs. Contraindications include coronary artery disease and uncontrolled hypertension. Triptans can be given by a variety of routes, e.g. oral, intranasal, or subcutaneous.

They act by being selective serotonin agonists (5HT1B/1D). Pharmacological action of triptans is related to their binding to serotonin 5-HT1B and 5-HT1D receptors in cranial blood vessels that causes constriction and subsequent inhibition of proinflammatory neuropeptide release. They are effective because they act on serotonin receptors in nerve endings as well as the blood vessels. This leads to a decrease in the release of several peptides, including calcitonin gene-related peptide (CGRP) and substance P. This prevents vasodilation induced by localized inflammation and relieves pain.

Pharmacokinetically, both long and short-acting drugs are available. Long acting is more effective during

Box 6.4: Available triptans.

- Sumatriptan (subcutaneous/nasal/oral)
- Almotriptan (oral)
- Eletriptan (oral)
- Frovatriptan (oral)
- Naratriptan (oral)
- Rizatriptan (oral)
- Zolmitriptan (oral).

Box 6.5: Triptans.

- *Short acting*:
  - Sumatriptan, almotriptan, rizatriptan, zolmitriptan, and eletriptan.
- *Longer half-lives*:
  - Naratriptan, frovatriptan.

aura but take longer to act. Short-acting drugs have more side effects. List of available triptans is given in Box 6.4.

Which triptan?

Recurrent headache may indicate need for repeat dose, not new triptans. Pharmacokinetics/dynamics profile is similar and so is the side effect profile. So, there is little to choose among them. Choice of triptans is given in Box 6.5.

Triptans are serotonin 5-HT1 agonists which reduce neurogenic inflammation. These are most effective if used at *onset of headache or aura,* though may be helpful at other phases. Importantly, triptans are used specifically for migraine. For nonresponders, one can try ergots (also act on norepinephrine, dopamine, or other receptors). They are generally well tolerated. Contraindications include uncontrolled hypertension, coronary artery disease, peripheral artery disease, cerebrovascular disease, and pregnancy. Hit and trials may be needed to determine the best triptan for a given patient.

Dihydroergotamine: Dihydroergotamine is a nonselective serotonin agonist that can be used by a variety of routes, e.g. nasal, subcutaneously, intramuscularly, or intravenously.

Contraindications include pregnancy (teratogenic) and with triptans. They are also contraindicated in coronary artery disease like triptans.

Adjutants: Antiemetics such as metoclopramide or ondansetron intravenously or given orally both as adjunct and monotherapy. Caffeine or steroids like dexamethasone or prednisone could be used as well.

Nasal Spray in Migraine

Several triptans have become available as nasal spray. One would have to administer them in each nostril, may repeat in 15 minutes. They work best if taken early. Longer half-life than sumatriptan, though not as reliable for some patients.

Rescue Drugs

Opiates are rarely used in migraine. They should be used only a few times per year if at all needed. Up to one-half of patients with recurrent headache do not adhere to drug treatment regimen due to side effects.

Prevention of Migraine

The NICE, UK recommends topiramate or propranolol in the prophylaxis of migraine. One has to be cautious about the use of both of these drugs in pregnancy. Gabapentin is not recommended for prophylaxis. Drugs for prophylaxis of migraine and their salient features are given in Box 6.6. Pharmacological doses and side effects are given in Table 6.2.

Box 6.6: Drugs for prophylaxis of migraine and their features.

- *Tricyclic antidepressants:* First line
  - Amitriptyline, doxepin, if sleep is disturbed.
- *Beta-blockers:* First line
  - Atenolol, nadolol.
- *Ca^{2+} channel blockers:* Less effective
  - Verapamil most commonly used.
- *Anticonvulsants:* Second line, valuable
  - Valproate and topiramate are quite effective
  - *Lamotrigine, levetiracetam:* No good data as yet
  - *Pregabalin:* It may help (anecdotal)
  - Psychotropic effects may be useful.
- *Ergots:* Rarely used for prevention
  - Side effects may be problematic
  - *Methysergide:* Fibrosis (use 6 months maximum).
- *Monoamine oxidase inhibitors:* Effective but have drawbacks
  - Tyramine-free diet a must
  - Numerous drug interactions.

TABLE 6.2: Common drugs of choice for migraine prophylaxis.

Drugs	*Dose*	*Side effects*
Beta blockers	–	–
Propranolol	40–420 mg	Bradycardia, bronchospasm, and fatigue
Metoprolol	100–200 mg	Bradycardia, fatigue
Atenolol	25–100 mg	Bradycardia, fatigue
Calcium channel blockers	–	–
Verapamil	80–320 mg	Bradycardia
Tricyclic antidepressants	–	–
Amitriptyline	10–100 mg	Dry mouth, sedation
Carbonic anhydrase inhibitor	–	Paresthesia, stone
Topiramate	25–100 mg	Paresthesia, stone

One should give prophylaxis when there is a disabling headache more than two times per month. Also, there is a poor relief from abortive therapy. Uncommon migraines, e.g. basilar or hemiplegic migraine need prophylaxis. One might also consider prophylaxis when there is a contraindication to acute therapy, e.g. coronary artery disease with migraine. Also failure of acute therapy could be one more indication. There could be several preferences for preventative therapy.

- *Antihypertensives*: All the drugs of antihypertensive class are effective. Best evidence for beta blockers is available and whole the evidence for calcium channels blockers is limited. Angiotensin-converting enzyme (ACE) inhibitors and angiotensin blockers are also effective. No evidence for diuretics is available.
- *Antidepressants*: Depression or other psychiatric disorder often comorbid conditions often coexist with migraine. Lack of evidence for selective serotonin reuptake inhibitors (SSRIs) exists but tricyclics and mirtazapine shown to have some benefit.
- *Anticonvulsants*: Sodium valproate is approved drug for migraine prophylaxis. It is at least as effective as beta blocker. The drug is well tolerated. Another drug from anticonvulsant class is topiramate. Weight loss benefit is there with topiramate. Gabapentin is not Food and Drug Administration (FDA) approved but appears to be effective.

Other Agents

Other agents include botulinum toxin injections have been tried. Coenzyme Q10 have shown benefits in small studies. Magnesium has shown mixed results.

Status migrainosus: Status migrainosus is prolonged (>72h), intractable migraine which is associated with nausea and vomiting.

MEDICATION OVERUSE HEADACHE[5]

Medication overuse headache is persistent, recurring headache in the setting of regular analgesics use. One should continue until medication is stopped. This type of headache is often responsible for "transformation" of episodic into chronic headache. Short-acting analgesic use more than 2–3 times/weeks. Headaches become predictable, more frequent, and even continuous with regular analgesics use in overdose. Medications no longer prevent headaches.

- Analgesics, especially short- or intermediate-acting, For example,
  - Opioids
  - Nonsteroidal anti-inflammatory drugs including acetaminophen
  - Combination analgesics
  - Caffeine
  - Triptans.

The NICE, UK recommends withdrawal of the analgesics as the preferred treatment.

TENSION HEADACHE[8]

This is a common cause of headache and is often episodic or chronic. It is important to know that it may be associated with possible migraine variant. Episodic form affects up to one-third of adults annually and less disability and morbidity than migraine may result.

The cause of tension headache is uncertain and perhaps involves activation of hyperexcitable peripheral afferent neurons from head and neck muscles. Associated muscle tenderness and psychological tension may aggravate the same. Abnormalities in central pain processing and generalized increased pain sensitivity are found in some individuals. Genetic factors may also play some role.

A typical "bandlike" like sensation may occur. The headache is bilateral, frontal, or temporoparietal. Referred (myofascial) pain from neck to head may occur. Neck structures may contribute to pain (*cervicogenic headache*).

International Headache Society criteria for tension headache are given here:

- At least 10 episodes fulfilling following criteria:
  - Headache lasting 30 minutes to 7 days
  - Has at least two of the following:
    - Bilateral location
    - Pressing/tightening (nonpulsating) quality
    - Mild or moderate intensity
    - Not aggravated by physical activity such as walking or climbing stairs.
  - No nausea or vomiting
  - Less than two episodes of photophobia or phonophobia
  - Not attributable to another disorder.

Management

Acute therapy for individual attacks include simple analgesics, e.g. aspirin 500–1,000 mg or other NSAIDs, e.g. paracetamol which is more effective than placebo but less effective than NSAIDs. Combination drugs containing simple analgesics and caffeine are helpful as well. Opioids or sedatives should not be used as impair alertness and can cause overuse and dependence.

Preventive treatment should be considered when headaches are frequent or acute attacks do not respond to abortive treatment. Preventive treatment can be considered when at least two episodes of headaches occur during a month.

Best evidence is for amitriptyline in dose of 25–150 mg/day. It helps both pain and muscle tenderness. Works best when started at low dose and increased weekly. Mirtazapine 15–30 mg/day could be other drug. SSRIs have not been found to be useful. Botulinum toxin has been tried with variable success.

Education, awareness, counseling, lifestyle, and nonpharmacological treatments, e.g. yoga, relaxation, etc. have little evidence to support or refute for tension type headache but can be recommended to individual case/s.

The NICE, UK guidelines advise NSAIDs as the primary form of treatment and forbid the use of opioids.

CLUSTER HEADACHE[9]

Cluster headache is a rare disorder and is seen more commonly in males. There is a genetic predisposition. Cluster headache comes in cycles/clusters lasting for weeks to months. Repetitive headaches during a cluster can occur; the headache may last for 1–3 hours apiece and is always unilateral.

Patients present with focal facial and eye pain, lacrimation, rhinorrhea, etc. This often occurs when sleeping or napping. A typical "cluster headache face", which is leonine face, furrowed and thickened skin with prominent folds, a broad chin, vertical forehead creases, and nasal telangiectasias can occur.

Management

The NICE, UK recommends 100% oxygen (12 liters/min via a rebreathing mask) or subcutaneous or nasal triptan as acute treatment options.

Drugs such as paracetamol, NSAIDs, opioids, or ergots/triptans given orally are not very effective.

Chronic/Preventive

The NICE, UK recommends lithium or verapamil for prophylaxis.

Other agents for prophylaxis are:

- Valproate
- Topiramate
- Prednisone
- Melatonin.

CHRONIC DAILY HEADACHE[10]

Chronic daily headache is a broad category consisting of chronic migraine, chronic tension-type headache, or new daily persistent headache. It generally has poor prognosis.

TRIGEMINAL NEURALGIA[11,12]

Trigeminal neuralgia is a disorder characterized by lancinating attacks of severe facial pain. Diagnosis based primarily on a history of characteristic pain attacks that are consistent with specific research and clinical criteria.

Trigeminal neuralgia is a brief (seconds to minutes) episodes of severe, sharp, stabbing, lancinating, pain, and is almost always unilateral. It is important to note that the bilateral facial pain could be suggestive of MS. Pain occurs along one or more trigeminal divisions. Spontaneous or evoked pain may have trigger zones. Multiple attacks may occur over short periods and patient may be asymptomatic between attacks. The facial sensations may be normal.

In majority of patients, clinical examination, imaging, and laboratory tests are unremarkable. In a smaller group, signs and symptoms secondary to another disease affecting the trigeminal system.

Box 6.7: Drugs in trigeminal neuralgia.

- *Antiepileptic drugs*:
  - Carbamazepine
  - Oxcarbazepine
  - Phenytoin
  - Gabapentin
  - Pregabalin
  - Lamotrigine
  - Topiramate
  - Tiagabine
  - Levetiracetam.
- *Tricyclic antidepressants*:
  - Amitriptyline
  - Nortriptyline
  - Desipramine.
- *Muscle relaxants*:
  - Baclofen.

Incidence is 4/100,000 and majority of cases are spontaneous but some familial cases reported too. Most cases are over the age of 50 years.

Antiepileptic drugs are the cornerstone of treatment and one would have to start low, titrate to relief or side effects. Also one should monitor side effects and drug interactions. Monitor levels and blood tests if indicated. Rotate other antiepileptic drugs or add as needed. Carbamazepine remains the gold standard. Response sometimes is so good that it was once thought to be diagnostic. Drugs used in the treatment of trigeminal neuralgia are given in Box 6.7.

Adverse effects of antiepileptic drugs used in trigeminal neuralgia include cognitive changes, e.g. sedation, nystagmus, ataxia, diplopia, dizziness, nausea, vomiting, headache, etc. Allergic reaction can occur with carbamazepine in some cases. There may be cross-sensitivity with phenytoin and carbamazepine. Phenytoin can cause gums enlargement, hirsutism, osteomalacia, etc.

Surgical Treatment of Trigeminal Neuralgia

Microvascular decompression or percutaneous ablative procedures like radiofrequency gangliolysis, glycerol rhizolysis, or balloon compression could be done. Stereotactic radiosurgery, e.g. gamma knife is popular now. Alcohol neurolysis was popular in the past.

CONCLUSION

Migraine, tension headache and cluster headaches are commonly encountered primary headaches. Secondary headaches account for 2% of headaches in general practice. Head trauma, vascular diseases, neoplasms, substance abuse or withdrawal, infection/inflammation, metabolic disorders, etc. are common reasons of secondary headaches.

First or worst headache (thunderclap headache), progressive or new daily persistent headaches, age >50 or <5 years, headaches associated with fever, rash, stiff neck and headaches associated with abnormal mental status or abnormal neurological examination may be warning signs.

Rule out potentially dangerous (secondary) headaches, e.g. Neoplasm, infection, hemorrhage, etc. Thorough history and physical examination is a must to diagnose headache types. One should implement treatment plan and monitor outcome.

REFERENCES

1. UpToDate. (2017). Patient education: Headache treatment in adults (beyond the basics). [online] Available from https://www.uptodate.com/contents/headache-treatment-in-adults-beyond-the-basics. [Accessed May, 2018].

2. Headache Australia. (2017). Headache management. [online] Available from http://headacheaustralia.org.au/headache-management/. [Accessed May, 2018].
3. National Institute for Health and Care Excellence (NICE). (2015). Headaches in over 12s: diagnosis and management. [online] Available from https://www.nice.org.uk/guidance/cg150. [Accessed May, 2018].
4. Huntington J, Yuan CL. Topiramate (Topamax) for migraine prophylaxis. Am Fam Physician. 2005;72(8): 1563-4.
5. WebMd. (2017). Migraine headache treatment. [online] Available from http://www.webmd.com/migraines-headaches/migraine-treatments#1. [Accessed May, 2018].
6. Migraine.com. (2017). Migraine treatment. [online] Available from https://migraine.com/migraine-treatment/. [Accessed May, 2018].
7. Chawla J. (2018). Migraine headache treatment and management. [online] Available from http://emedicine.medscape.com/article/1142556-treatment. [Accessed May, 2018].
8. Blanda M. (2017). Cluster headache treatment and management. [online] Available from http://emedicine.medscape.com/article/1142459-treatment. [Accessed May, 2018].
9. National Health Trust Choices. (2015). Tension-type headaches. [online] Available from https://www.nhs.uk/conditions/tension-headaches/. [Accessed May, 2018].
10. Mayo Clinic. (2017). Chronic daily headaches. [online] Available from https://www.mayoclinic.org/diseases-conditions/chronic-daily-headaches/diagnosis-treatment/drc-20370897. [Accessed May, 2018].
11. National Health Trust Choices (NHS). (2016). Trigeminal neuralgia. [online] Available from https://www.nhs.uk/conditions/trigeminal-neuralgia/treatment/. [Accessed May, 2018].
12. Facial Pain Association. (2017). Treatment options for trigeminal neuralgia. [online] Available from http://fpa-support.org/learn/treatment-options/. [Accessed May, 2018].

CHAPTER

7

Myasthenia Gravis

INTRODUCTION

Myasthenia gravis is fluctuating weakness increased by exertion. The weakness increases during the day and improves with rest. Extraocular muscle weakness is usually the presenting feature; so the patients may first be seen by ophthalmologists rather than neurologists. Ptosis is present initially in half of patients and during the course of disease in almost all of the patients. Head extension and flexion weakness can occur and weakness may be worse in proximal muscles. Progression of disease may be slow in mild disease and may take weeks to months. Usually the disease spreads from ocular to facial to bulbar to truncal and limb muscles.[1] Antibodies to receptors are responsible for muscle weakness (Fig. 7.1).

Often, symptoms may remain limited to extraocular muscles and eyelid muscles for years. The disease remains ocular in one-seventh of patients. Spontaneous remissions are rare and most remissions with treatment occur within the first 3 years.[2]

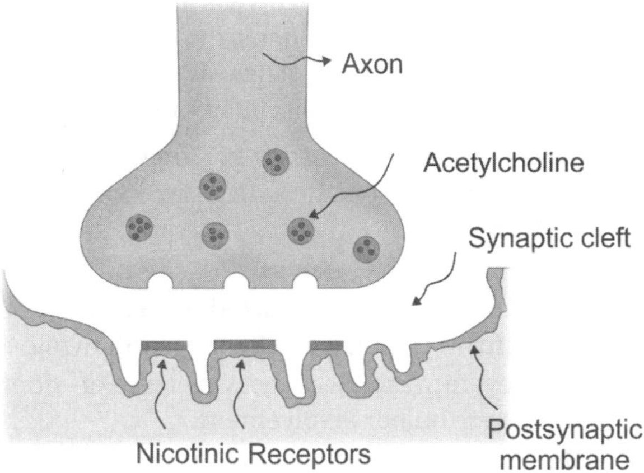

Fig. 7.1: Neuromuscular junction. The pathophysiology of myasthenia gravis involves the presence of antibodies to nicotinic receptors.

DIAGNOSIS[3,4]

Myasthenia gravis is a disease of skeletal muscle acetylcholine receptors, where antinicotinic receptor antibodies develop at neuromuscular junctions. The chemical transmitter, acetylcholine (ACh) is unable to bind to the receptors (AChR) on the postsynaptic membrane to transmit the nerve impulse to muscle fibers to produce a muscle contraction.

Intermittent diplopia can be presenting feature of myasthenia gravis. Frequent purchases of new glasses to correct blurry vision, difficulty focusing and/or early onset of convergence insufficiency of a need for prism correction could be another features. Use of dark glasses to reduce diplopia or hide drooping eyelids is seen sometimes.

Avoidance of certain foods that become difficult to chew and swallow or cessation of activities that require prolonged use of muscle activity, e.g. jogging/walking, etc.

Because the majority of patients with myasthenia gravis present with ocular manifestations, the ophthalmologist plays an essential role in the diagnosis of this condition and a high index of suspicion facilitates the diagnosis.

Clinical classification of myasthenia gravis:

i. Ocular manifestations alone (e.g. diplopia, dropping of eyelids).

iia. Mild generalized weakness.

iib. Moderately severe generalized weakness + some bulbar involvement, e.g. difficulty swallowing.

iii. Acute severe muscle weakness over weeks–months with severe bulbar involvement.

iv. Late severe with marked bulbar involvement.

Edrophonium/Tensilon Test

Patients with myasthenia gravis have low numbers of acetylcholine receptor (AChR) at the neuromuscular junction. Ach released from the motor nerve terminal is metabolized by acetylcholine esterase enzyme, a quick enzyme that can degrade Ach really fast.

Edrophonium is a short-acting acetylcholinesterase inhibitor that improves muscle weakness. One should evaluate weakness (i.e. ptosis and ophthalmoplegia) before and after administration.

TREATMENT[5-11]

Anticholinesterase inhibitors are the mainstay of treatment. Pyridostigmine is the drug of choice. The drug starts working in 30–60 minutes and lasts for 3–6 hours; so repeat doses are needed. One would have to individualize doses. Adult dose is typically 60–300 mg/daily orally or 2 mg intravenous (IV)/intramuscular (IM) every 2–3 hours is usual dose. Caution is to check for cholinergic crisis. Other drugs include neostigmine.

IMMUNOMODULATING THERAPIES[6-11]

Prednisone

This is the most commonly used corticosteroid. Significant improvement is often seen after a decreased antibody titer which is usually 1–4 months.

Prednisone 60–80 mg/day given until sustained improvement (usually 2 weeks) then alternate days beginning with 100–120 mg tapered over months to lowest dose necessary (usually less than 20 mg alternate days).

Improvement or complete relief of symptoms occurs in 75% of cases. Improvement in first 6–8 weeks, but strength may increase to total remission over months.

Patients with thymoma have an excellent response to prednisone before or after thymectomy.

No single dose regimens is accepted as some start low and go high and others start high dose to achieve a quicker response. Clearance may be decreased by estrogens or digoxin. Patients taking concurrent diuretics should be monitored for hypokalemia.

DIET IN MYASTHENIA GRAVIS[12]

- Patients may experience difficulty in chewing and swallowing due to oropharyngeal weakness.
- If dysphagia develops, liquids should be thickened as thick liquids decrease risk for aspiration.

PHYSICAL ACTIVITY IN MYASTHENIA GRAVIS

- Patients should be advised to be as active as possible but should rest frequently and avoid sustained activity.
- One should educate patients about fluctuating nature of weakness and exercise-induced fatigability.

CONCLUSION

Treatment goals must be individualized according to the severity of the disease, the patient's age and sex, and the degree of functional impairment. The response to any form of treatment is difficult to access because the severity of symptoms fluctuates. Spontaneous improvement, even remissions, occur without specific therapy, especially during the early stages of the disease. That however should not be taken for granted. In an individual case, the treatment of myasthenia gravis can be challenging; more so in primary care setting.

REFERENCES

1. Jowkar A (2018). Myasthenia gravis. [online] Available from https://emedicine.medscape.com/article/1171206-overview. [Accessed May, 2018].
2. Mayo Clinic. (2017). Myasthenia gravis. [online] Available from https://www.mayoclinic.org/diseases-conditions/myasthenia-gravis/symptoms-causes/syc-20352036. [Accessed May, 2018].
3. MedicineNet.com (2017). Facts, treatment and tests of myasthenia gravis. [online] Available from https://www.medicinenet.com/myasthenia_gravis/article.htm. [Accessed May, 2018].
4. Sanders DB, Wolfe GI, Benatar M, et al. (2016). International consensus guidance for management of myasthenia gravis: Executive summary. [online] Available from http://n.neurology.org/content/neurology/early/2016/06/29/WNL.0000000000002790.full.pdf. [Accessed May, 2018].
5. Sussman J, Farrugia ME, Maddison P, et al. Myasthenia gravis: Association of British Neurologists' management guidelines. Pract Neurol. 2015;15(3):199-206.
6. National Institute for Health and Care Excellence (2017). Myasthenia gravis. [online] Available from https://www.evidence.nhs.uk/search?q=myasthenia+gravis+and+management. [Accessed May, 2018].

7. Bird SJ (2017). Treatment of myasthenia gravis. [online] Available from https://www.uptodate.com/contents/treatment-of-myasthenia-gravis. [Accessed May, 2018].
8. American Academy of Neurology (AAN) (2017). Neuromuscular diseases. [online] Available from https://www.aan.com/Guidelines/Home/ByTopic?topicId=19. [Accessed May, 2018].
9. Liu WB, Ran H, Ou CY, et al. Developing an international consensus guidance for myasthenia gravis using RAND/UCLA appropriateness method. Neuroimmunol Neuroinflammation. 2017;4:54-60.
10. Gilhus NE, Owe JF, Hoff JM, et al. Myasthenia gravis: a review of available treatment approaches. Autoimmune Dis. 2011;2011:847393.
11. Gilhus NE. Myasthenia gravis. N Engl J Med. 2016;375:2570-81.
12. Turner C. A review of myasthenia gravis: Pathogenesis, clinical features and treatment. Curr Anesth Crit Care. 2007;18(1):15-23.

CHAPTER

8

Drug Treatment of Movement Disorders

INTRODUCTION

Movement disorders are common[1] with varied presentation. Given here are two examples for better understanding:

Case 1

A young boy of 8 years old has a history of allergic rhinitis unresponsive to nasal steroids. The patient has 1 year history of recurrent neck popping, multiple times daily. There is loss of consciousness and is aware of movements. Patient says that he feels "relaxed" after movements. What is the diagnosis and what comorbidities should be inquired into? Does he really have rhinitis?

Case 2

A young kid of 6 years old (female child) presents in emergency department with abnormal sustained twisting posture of left arm and neck. There have been few recent visits for headache with vomiting in the past. The patient has taken headache medicine for the last 5 days. There are no other medications that the patient has taken. There is no other significant history. What is the diagnosis and what is treatment?

EVALUATION[1-3]

One would have to start by knowing if the movements are normal or abnormal? One should also see if they paroxysmal (sudden on/off), continual (repeated again and again), or continuous (nonstop)? How does voluntary movement affect abnormal movements? Are movements present at rest, posture, action, intention, or combination? An important point is that if the environmental stimuli/emotion precipitate/exacerbate/alleviate?

Additionally, one can ascertain if the patient aware of movements or not? Do movements stop with sleep? Box 8.1 given here gives details of the types of commonly occurring movements.

Box 8.1: Commonly seen abnormal movements.

- *Hyperkinetic (most common)*:
  - Tic
  - Tremor
  - Myoclonus
  - Chorea
  - Ballismus
  - Athetosis
  - Dystonia
  - Dyskinesia
  - Akathisia
  - Myokymia
  - Asterixis.
- *Hypokinetic*:
  - Bradykinesia
  - Freezing
  - Rigidity.

DYSTONIA

Dystonia is the presence of abnormal twisting movement sustained for a long time. Dyskinesia as a term may be applied to any involuntary movement, although commonly used to refer to induced chorea and dystonia.

Spasticity and hyperkinetic are two main types of dystonias. Blepharospasm, craniocervical (Meige) and oromandibular are commonly seen type of dystonias. Tardive dyskinesia and Wilson's disease are other examples.

Drug-induced (e.g. D2 blockers), psychogenic and toxins/metabolic are other causes.

Dystonias are treated by a number of treatment options:

- Anticholinergics (e.g. trihexyphenidyl)
- Dopamine agonists or levodopa (if dopa sensitive)
- GABA agonists ($GABA_A$ like benzodiazepines and $GABA_B$ like baclofen, also intrathecal)
- Botulinum toxins
- Surgical (Myectomy, DBS, thalamotomy, etc.).

TICS

The Taskforce on Childhood Movement Disorders defines, "tics are repeated, individually recognizable, intermittent movements or movement fragments that are almost always briefly suppressible and are usually associated with awareness of an urge to perform the movement".

Sometimes, it is difficult for young children to describe urge. Dystonic movements disappear with sleep and are often worsened by anxiety. Transient tic disorder may affect children and tics last less than 1 year. Chronic tic disorder involves tics that last more than 1 year. Tourette's syndrome involves chronic tics with both motor and vocal tics.

Gilles de la Tourette syndrome is rare disorders with tics as major clinical manifestation. The condition has with associated behavioral disorders present in about 1% patients. Combination of motor and vocal tics are present. The disease has its beginning in childhood. Attention deficit hyperactivity disorder, obsessive-compulsive disorder and impulsiveness are present.

TREMORS

Tremors are rhythmic oscillation around a central point involving one or more body parts. Different tremors occur at different times—rest, postural, action, and intention. Table 8.1 gives details of the types of tremors.

Treatment

Treatment is usually started with beta blockers, e.g. propranolol. The starting treatment is 10 mg twice daily to increase in the dose to 20 mg twice daily within a week. Fatigue, bradycardia, impotence, and bronchospasm may occur.

Primidone, a prodrug of phenobarbitone is not available in India but can be started at 12.5 mg per day and increased to 50 mg twice daily. In some patients, higher dose is needed.

Other drugs like alprazolam (0.25–3 mg daily) or lorazepam (1–10 mg daily) could also be used. Zonisamide in doses 100 mg daily increased to 200 mg daily could be used.

CHOREA

Chorea is the presence of chaotic, purposeless movements. These are not as rapid as myoclonus. Chorea type

TABLE 8.1: Types of tremors.

Types	*Diagnosis*
Resting tremor	Parkinson's disease
Postural tremor	Physiologic tremor, essential tremor
Intention tremor	Cerebellar disease

movements can be seen in CP, Sydenham, postpump, kernicterus, hereditary, etc. Ballism is large amplitude chorea of proximal muscles which may be violent also.

Chorea involves irregular, random movements of body parts, usually quick, twisting, with distal predominance, etc. The disease involves corpus striatum (e.g. caudatus, putamen). *Pharmacological mechanism includes a* hyperdopaminergic state. *Standard pharmacological treatment consists of* neuroleptics. Chorea can occur in a variety of conditions and disorders. Chorea may be the presenting feature of Huntington's disease, and other progressive neurological disorders. It may also be caused by drugs (levodopa, antipsychotics), by metabolic disorders, endocrine disorders, and vascular lesions.

DYSTONIA

The Task Force on dystonia defines "a movement disorder in which involuntary sustained or intermittent muscle contractions cause twisting and repetitive movements, abnormal postures, or both". Dystonic postures are repeated, particular patterns or postures are characteristic of any one patient at a given time. Postures may be sustained or occur during brief intervals. Some dystonic postures are often triggered by certain voluntary movements, e.g. writer's cramps.

Dystonis is the sustained muscle contractions producing twisting and repetitive movements or abnormal postures of affected body parts. Striatum, pallidum, thalamus and their connections are involved. *Pharmacological mechanism leading to dystonia involve* hypercholinergic and hypodopaminergic states. *Standard pharmacological treatments* are anti-cholinergics.

National Health Trust, UK recommends four main treatments for dystonia:

1. Botulinum toxin
2. Drugs
3. Physiotherapy
4. Surgery like deep brain stimulation.

Common treatment involves using botulinum toxin, levodopa, or clonazepam and trihexyphenidyl. The drugs like clonazepam boost activity of gamma-aminobutyric acid and anticholinergic drugs like trihexyphenidyl, biperiden, or procyclidine reduce cholinergic activity. Some levodopa responsive dystonia may have dramatic response to these drugs. Tetrabenazine, a dopamine depletory could also be used.

Tetrabenazine

Tetrabenazine is a neuron depletor that inhibits vesicular monoamine transporter-2. Typical starting dose is 6.25 mg given twice daily and effective dose is 25 mg given twice. Metabolism of the drug is affected by CYP2D6 polymorphism. The drug is FDA approved for Huntington's chorea and is also effective for tardive dyskinesia and some dystonias. Sedation and mental depression are major side effects.

Botulinum Toxin

Botulinum toxin inhibits presynaptic Ach release by destroying SNARE proteins. Dosing can be tricky in an individual patient. The drug is an FDA approved for cervical dystonia, blepharospasm, and a few other disorders. Typical duration of action is 90–120 days. Skeletal muscle weakness is the major side effects.

ATHETOSIS

Athetosis is slow, continuous, and writhing movements of distal body parts, especially fingers and hands. Athetosis can be seen in cerebral palsy and Rett syndrome.[4]

MYOCLONUS[5,6]

Myoclonus is sudden, brief, and shock-like movements, which may be repetitive or rhythmic.

Myoclonus is short synchronous monophasic muscle jerks (agonists and antagonists in the same region), of irregular frequency and amplitude. This could be epileptic or nonepileptic. According to distribution of signs; it could be focal, segmentary or generalised. In terms of location, it can be cortical, subcortical (reticular, brainstem) or spinal.

STEREOTYPIES

The Task Force defines, "stereotypies are repetitive, simple movements that can be voluntarily suppressed". These are patterned, episodic, repetitive, and purposeless movements that are different from tics, and are seen often in autism, Rett syndrome.

BENIGN MOVEMENT DISORDERS

Benign neonatal sleep myoclonus and benign myoclonus of infancy are examples of benign movement disorders.

TOURETTE SYNDROME

This is not an uncommon disorder with chronic vocal and motor tics. Comorbidities include attention deficit hyperkinetic disorder, obsessive compulsive disorder, and anxiety often guides treatment.

Treatment

This is only needed if there is physical discomfort, functional problems, or psychosocial problems. Alpha-adrenergic drugs such as clonidine, selective serotonin reuptake inhibitor (SSRI), antiepileptics, e.g. topiramate or levetiracetam could be used. One can use antipsychotics but may have higher side-effect profile (e.g. haloperidol).

SYDENHAM'S CHOREA[7]

This is the most common form of acquired chorea in childhood. Usually it occurs 1–18 months after group A beta-hemolytic streptococci infection (contrast to carditis and arthritis that appear within 1 month). This form of chorea can also have emotional change (deteriorating school performance), psychiatric symptoms—obsessive compulsive disorder, irritability, and hypotonia. Grip-strength testing has continuous increase/decrease, commonly called as milking sign. Work-up includes electrocardiogram/echocardiography (ECG/echo) to look for carditis, antistreptolysin O (ASO) titers, and Dnase B antibodies. Other causes of chorea, e.g. systemic lupus erythematosus (SLE), Huntington's disease, encephalitis, and Wilson's disease should be ruled out.

Treatment

Antiepileptics like valproic acid or carbamazepine are effective in reducing choreiform movements. Steroids are widely used. Dopaminergic blocking drugs, e.g. haloperidol could be effective. Prednisolone, intravenous immunoglobulin (IVIG), or plasma exchange therapy could be used.

Treatment involves dose penicillin for 10 days, followed by antibiotic prophylaxis against group A beta-hemolytic streptococci. Specific treatment may be needed, e.g. divalproex sodium, phenobarbital, haldol, pimozide, valium, and carbamazepine. Steroids may shorten duration.

Wilson's Disease

Wilson's disease occurs as a result of excessive copper accumulation due to mutation of the ATP7B gene. Low ceruloplasmin and high urine copper are seen. Kayser-Fleischer rings are the hallmark physical signs. The disease affects liver, bone, and behavior.

Treatment consists of using copper chelators, e.g. penicillamine or trientine in the acute phase. In the long-term phase, use of zinc, low copper diet and liver transplant can be considered.

OPSOCLONUS-MYOCLONUS SYNDROME

Dancing eyes or dancing feet may indicate opsoclonus-myoclonus syndrome. The mean age of onset is 2 years.

Opsoclonus is uncontrolled, frequent, conjugate, and saccadic movement of eyes in all directions. These patients can also have ataxia [opsoclonus-myoclonus-ataxia (OMA)], irritability, sleep problems, etc.

Causes include autoimmune, e.g. paraneoplastic—neuroblastoma (unknown antibody) or parainfectious, etc.

Early and sufficient immunotherapy can ensure neurological remission. If tumor is present, then surgical correction is indicated. One can treat movements with immunosuppression—steroids, IVIG, or rituximab. Almost all patients can show some degree of improvement over this.

RETT SYNDROME[8-11]

Rett syndrome is an X-linked dominant and is mostly sporadic. The condition occurs almost exclusively in girls. Mutations in *MECP2* gene on Xq28 and is a rare syndrome.

Typical presentation includes a female baby at 6–18 months with previously normal growth and development with regression in verbal and motor skills. Postnatal microcephaly can occur. Baby may purposeful movements of hands or stereotypies of hands resembling hand washing and kneading. Differential diagnoses include autism, cerebellopontine angle tumor, Fragile X-syndrome, Angelman syndrome, leukodystrophies, neurocutaneous syndromes, metabolic disorders, etc.

Treatment

There are standard available treatments for Rett syndrome. However, good medical care and symptomatic medications can be supportive. Physical therapy could improve outlook. Good nutrition, behavioral therapy, speech, and occupational therapy could be done.

PARKINSON'S DISEASE[12,13]

This is a major movement disorder. Tremor, rigidity, bradykinesia (slowness of movement), and postural impairment are presenting symptoms.

Onset of disease occurs after 60 years and the course may run for 10–25 years. Males are affected more than females and there is some genetic predisposition. Predisposing factors are given here in Box 8.2.

Tremor is present in majority of patients and is 4–6 Hz resting tremor (*pill rolling*). It is usually by voluntary activity, by stress.

Rigidity is increased resistance to passive movements (*cogwheel rigidity*). There is no muscle weakness or change in deep tendon reflexes.

Slowness of movements is a prominent symptom and often patients report this by themselves. It may be noticed in speech as well as in voluntary movements.

Box 8.2: Predisposing factors.

- Positive family history
- Male gender
- Pesticide exposure
- Head trauma.

Difficulty with balance and gait occurs late in the course of disease and its occurrence in early part of disease should suggest alternative diagnosis.

Loss of melanin-containing dopaminergic neurons in substantia nigra seems to be a major responsible factor. Lewy bodies—protein balls in the neurons are pathological hallmark of Parkinson's disease (PD) in basal ganglia.

Diagnosis is clinical and there is no particular laboratory test or biomarker. By the time symptoms appear, dopamine depletion may have occurred by 80%.

Treatment

Goal of Treatment

There is no proven clinically neuroprotective drug that can halt the progression of PD. The treatment should be started when functional disability starts. The goal is to maintain function and quality of life and avoid drug-induced complications.

Levodopa

- Levodopa is considered to be the gold standard treatment. The drug is used in combination with carbidopa.[12] It is a prodrug that gets converted to dopamine in brain. Dopamine itself cannot cross blood/brain barrier so a precursor is needed. The drug improves *all* features of PD, but wears off over time.
- Levodopa has been the first line for years, but now primarily *second line* due to side effects such as on and off phenomena. There are some hypothetical concerns also that free radicals generated by the

oxidative metabolism of dopamine contribute further to the degeneration of dopaminergic neurons. However, there is no direct proof for the same.

- Nausea, vomiting, and wearing off—when effects of single dose do not last as long as it used to last. Dyskinesias—sudden, uncontrollable, and jerky movements of arms, legs, head, and trunk can occur. On/off response—due to fluctuating levels of dopa can occur. During the "on phase", there may be uncontrolled movements and during "off phase", there may be ↓ motion and freezing episodes may occur.
- Levodopa is often given in association with carbidopa—(decarboxylase inhibitor). In advanced patients, it is given with entacapone which is a catechol-O-methyltransferase (COMT) inhibitor working by inhibiting the breakdown of catecholamines and prolongs half-life of levodopa. The purpose is to decreased levodopa breakdown/conversion in bloodstream, maximizes delivery to brain, and minimizes nausea. Dosing should start with one 25/100 mg carbidopa/levodopa tablet three times a day.

Anticholinergics

- Drugs like trihexyphenidyl are commonly used as anticholinergics in young onset PD patients. Other alternatives include benztropine, orphenadrine, procyclidine, and biperiden.
- Trihexyphenidyl is the usual starting drug but is tolerated poorly by elderly. They are the oldest class of drugs but are avoided in patients with prostatic enlargement, glaucoma, constipation, or urinary retention.

Dopamine Agonists

- *Dopamine agonists may offer some degree of neuroprotection and have reduced risk of motor fluctuations.*

- Bromocriptine, pergolide, pramipexole, ropinirole, and apomorphine—injectable, rapid-acting, "rescue" drug for acute freezing episodes. Side effect includes severe nausea and vomiting.
- Dopamine agonists such as ropinirole and pramipexole behave like dopamine by stimulating dopamine receptor directly. They can be used as initial monotherapy to preserve use of dopamine for later in disease course. Dopamine agonists can also be used as add-on to dopamine when levodopa alone is no longer effective or side effects have become intolerable. Side effect includes sudden-onset sleepiness akin to narcolepsy or sleep attacks.

Amantadine

- Amantadine is basically a short-acting antiviral flu drug, which also has antidyskinetic properties for mild symptoms. The mechanism of action is unclear but probably is related to its dopamine facilitation.
- Side effects include restlessness, confusion, rash, edema, nausea, and cardiac arrhythmias. Ankle edema is common side effect and is treated by diuretics.

Monoamine Oxidase Inhibitors

- Monoamine oxidase type B inhibitor such as selegiline, rasagiline acts by decreasing levodopa breakdown and may decrease dopamine reuptake. Selegiline is indicated in young onset PD patients and the drug is used for its modest effects for mild symptoms and it reduces "off" time. It may be neuroprotective. Side effects include confusion, nausea, headache, and insomnia. The risk of motor fluctuations is reduced when they are started early. The disability is also reduced and so is the need of levodopa.[13]

- As per American Association of Family Physicians treatment with monoamine oxidase-B inhibitors, amantadine or anticholinergics like trihexyphenidyl may modestly improve mild symptoms; however, most patients may need levodopa or a dopamine agonist in the later course of disease.[13]

CONCLUSION

Parkinsonism is the major movement disorder and is a disease of old age. Spasticity is common in children and tics are common in neuropsychiatric conditions. Cataplexy/Drop attacks could be surprising cause of sudden reduced movements. Hypothyroidism or other endocrinological disorders could be reasons behind hypokinesis. Hesitant gait of older individuals should be interpreted with caution. Tremors are most common type of hyperkinesis disorders and chorea, dystonic movements, myoclonus, ataxia and dysmetria are seen as a part of many neurological diseases. Akathisia is common in many psychiatric diseases. Restless legs or periodic hypnogogic movements could represent diagnostic confusion. Management consists of establishing proper diagnosis and treating symptomatically.

REFERENCES

1. Vanderbilt Health (2017). Movement disorders. [online] Available from www.mc.vanderbilt.edu/documents/.../files/Movement%20Disorders%20Babcock.ppt. [Accessed May, 2018].
2. International Parkinson and Movement Disorder Society (2017). Movement disorder. [online] Available from https://www.movementdisorders.org/MDS.htm. [Accessed May, 2018].
3. Johns Hopkins Medicine (2017). Types of movement disorders. [online] Available from https://www.hopkinsmedicine.org/neurology_neurosurgery/centers_

clinics/movement_disorders/conditions/index.html. [Accessed May, 2018].

4. WebMD. (2017). Rett syndrome: What to know. [online] Available from https://www.webmd.com/brain/autism/rett-syndrome#2. [Accessed May, 2018].
5. Bernstein BE (2017). Rett syndrome treatment and management. [online] Available from https://emedicine.medscape.com/article/916377-treatment. [Accessed May, 2018].
6. National Organization for Rare Disorders (NORD) (2017). Opsoclonus-myoclonus syndrome. [online] Available from https://rarediseases.org/rare-diseases/opsoclonus-myoclonus-syndrome/. [Accessed May, 2018].
7. Langille MM. (2015). Chorea in children. [online] Available from https://emedicine.medscape.com/article/1181993-overview#a4. [Accessed May, 2018].
8. WebMD. (2017). Dystonia: causes, types, symptoms, and treatments. [online] Available from https://www.webmd.com/brain/dystonia-causes-types-symptoms-and-treatments#2. [Accessed May, 2018].
9. The Dystonia Society (2017). Drugs used for dystonia. [online] Available from https://www.dystonia.org.uk/drugs-used-for-dystonia. [Accessed May, 2018].
10. National Health Trust (2017). Dystonia treatment choices. [online] Available from https://www.nhs.uk/conditions/dystonia/. [Accessed May, 2018].
11. Pal PK. Guidelines for management of essential tremor. Ann Indian Acad Neurol. 2011;14(Suppl 1):S25-8.
12. Hauser RA (2018). Parkinson disease treatment and management. [online] Available from https://emedicine.medscape.com/article/1831191-treatment. [Accessed May, 2018].
13. Rao SS, Hofmann LA, Shakil A. Parkinson's disease: diagnosis and treatment. Am Fam Physician. 2006;74(12):2046-54.

CHAPTER

9

Drug Treatment of Neurodegenerative Disease

NEURODEGENERATION[1]

What is Degeneration?

Neurodegenerative diseases are a group of disorders that share similar general clinical and pathological characteristics.

Many neurodegenerative diseases were considered idiopathic in the past that have been found to have specific etiology, e.g. inherited or familial. Basic pathogenetic mechanism of cell death is either apoptosis or degeneration. The diseases have insidious onset.

The diseases are progressive, however, with relentless clinical course. No apparent evoking factor may be present. Selective involvement of neuronal systems that are anatomically or physiologically related can occur. There are several examples of such diseases (Box 9.1), some of which are described elsewhere while the rest are detailed here.

Box 9.1: Common neurodegenerative diseases.

- Alzheimer's disease
- Parkinson's disease
- Amyotrophic lateral sclerosis
- Huntington's disease
- Friedreich's ataxia
- Spinal muscular atrophy.

Diagnosis

Diagnosis is made clinically and radiologically showing atrophy in various areas such as posterior cerebrum, hippocampus, or entorhinal area.

DEMENTIA[2-4]

Dementia is the acquired loss of cognitive abilities. There are several types of dementias. Alzheimer's disease (AD) (Fig. 9.1) is by far the most common type. Other common types of dementias are given in Box 9.2.

Alzheimer's Disease[2,3]

Worldwide, about 5–10% of people over the age of 65 years are affected and the number doubles every 5 years over age of 65 years → 50% in over 80 years.

Alzheimer's disease is also known as senile dementia of the Alzheimer type or simply AD. It is by far the most common form of dementia. This incurable, degenerative, and terminal disease was first described by a German psychiatrist and neuropathologist Alois Alzheimer in 1906 and was named after him.

Alzheimer's disease is a slowly progressive disease of the brain that is characterized by impairment of memory and eventually by disturbances in reasoning, planning, language, and perception. The disease begins by minor forgetfulness that progress to severe one and deterioration of personality.

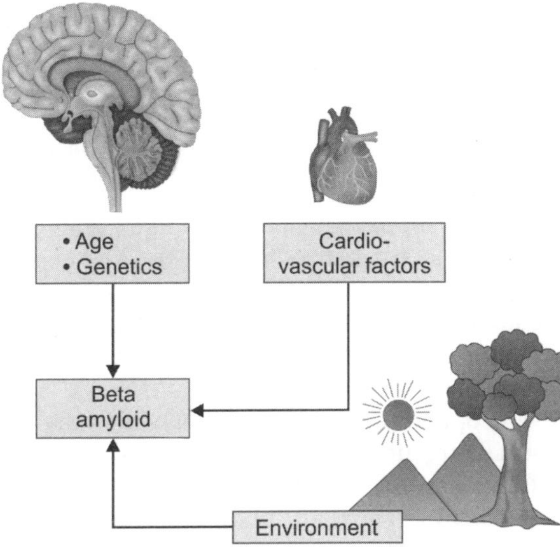

Fig. 9.1: Pathophysiology of the most common type of dementia, i.e. Alzheimer's disease. Age and genetics are major factors, while the supportive role is played by cardiovascular (e.g. diabetes, hypertension) and environmental factors. Depression and lack of sleep too are associated with high frequency of dementia.

Box 9.2: Common types of dementias.

- Alzheimer's disease
- Frontotemporal dementia
- Vascular dementia
- Parkinson's disease with dementia
- Lewy body dementia
- Progressive supranuclear palsy (PSP)
- Normal pressure hydrocephalus
- Creutzfeldt-Jakob disease
- Huntington's disease.

Pathology

The two most significant physical findings in AD are: (1) neuritic plaques and (2) neurofibrillary tangles. It is, however, not clear if these cause or the result of the disease process.

Treatment[4]

One should rule out reversible dementia before proceeding with the treatment of dementias (*see* below).

Reversible dementias:

- Medications (e.g. benzodiazepines)
- Alcohol
- Metabolic (B12 deficiency, thyroid, hyponatremia, hypercalcemia, hepatic and renal dysfunction)
- Depression
- CNS neoplasms, chronic subdural hematoma
- Normal pressure hydrocephalous.

  Patients should be cautioned against unrealistic expectations from anticholinesterase drugs or other drugs used in dementias as they cannot cure dementias. One should also watch for return of insight leading to depression or anxiety, which may occur during course of therapy in some patients. Stopping of drugs may be needed in patients with unacceptable side effects, lack of response to medication and late stages of the disease.
- *Cholinesterase inhibitors*: Although there is currently no way to cure AD or stop its progression, encouraging advances in Alzheimer's treatment have been done, including drugs and nondrug approaches to improve symptom management. Cholinesterase inhibitors have been the traditionally successful approach. These act to increase the levels of acetylcholine in the brain, which plays a key role in memory and learning. This kind of drug postpones the worsening of symptoms for about a year in about half of the people. Cholinesterase inhibitors have traditionally been used for mild to moderate AD and include donepezil, rivastigmine, and galantamine, etc. However, in

recent times, rivastigmine and donepezil have been approved for all grades of severity of dementia.

Table-Goals of treatment of dementias:

- Cure disease (e.g. Vitamin B12 and thyroid deficiency dementias)
- Prevent disease or delay onset
- Slow down progression of disease
- Treat primary symptoms, e.g. memory deficits
- Treat secondary symptoms, e.g. depression/hallucinations, etc.

Cholinesterase inhibitors are indicated upon specialist diagnosis of Alzheimer's Disease, and a MMSE score of 10 to 24. An improvement on MMSE may be hard to see but patients could be seen as 'stabilized' for sometimes on these medications. Dramatic responses could occasionally be seen. Side effects such as nausea, vomiting, diarrhea, dizziness, headache, muscle cramps could be dose limiting side effects. One should use them carefully if gastric ulcer, heart disease, chronic lung disease/asthma are present.

Patients should be cautioned against unrealistic expectations from anticholinesterase drugs as they cannot cure dementias. One should also watch for return of insight leading to depression or anxiety, which may occur during course of therapy in some patients. Stopping of drugs may be needed in patients with unacceptable side effects, lack of response to medication and late stages of the disease.

- *Tacrine*: Tacrine is the oldest cholinesterase inhibitor in clinical use. One systematic review with more than 1,000 patients had demonstrated its clinical efficacy. Clinically insignificant improvement in cognition has been noted in clinical studies. Significant risk of liver function tests abnormalities have been detected hence, it is no more used clinically.

- *Donepezil*: This is the most commonly used cholinesterase inhibitor clinically. The drug acts by enhancing cholinergic function and increasing the concentration of acetylcholine by the virtue of inhibition of acetylcholinesterase.
  The advantages include easy titration (start 5 mg/day, then 10 mg after 4 weeks). A 23 mg long-acting formulation has been approved for treatment of severe dementia of Alzheimer's type. The side effects are gastrointestinal, e.g. nausea, diarrhea, cramps, etc. Some patients may have bradycardia, sleep alterations, and hallucinations.
- *Rivastigmine*: Rivastigmine is another anti-cholinesterase drug available to treat dementia of Alzheimer's type or Parkinson's disease dementia (PDD). The drug is available in the form of capsules (1.5–6 mg) or patches (5–15 mg/ cm^2, actual dose = 9.5–13.3 mg/24 h). The drug is approved for all grades of severity of dementia. No dose adjustment is needed in renal failure but may be needed in hepatic failure. Allergic reactions to patches may occur in some cases; rests of side effects are similar to donepezil (e.g. nausea, vomiting, diarrhea, loss of appetite, etc.).

• *Glutamate receptor antagonists*: Memantine has been approved for moderate-to-severe disease. Memantine can be used alone or in combination with acetylcholinesterase inhibitors like donepezil. Side effects include headache, constipation, confusion, and dizziness. The drug is used in dose of 5 mg twice daily, increased to 10 mg twice daily after 4 weeks. Dose in severe renal failure needs to be reduced to half; however, in liver disease, dose adjustments are not needed.

• *Antidepressants*: Drugs like selective serotonin reuptake inhibitors (SSRIs) help concomitant (early) depression. Drugs of SSRI class have no effect on cognitive function. Tricyclic antidepressants with significant anticholinergic functions need to be avoided though.

It is important to note that there is no long-term safety/efficacy data to support any significant benefit for treating behavioral symptoms of dementia with antipsychotic agents on regular basis. Small group of patients with active psychoses, disturbing hallucinations, or aggressive behaviors may have some benefits with antipsychotic drugs (e.g. olanzapine 5 mg/risperidone 0.5 to 2 mg on as per needed basis).

Side effects such as sedation, anticholinergic effects, Prolonged QT interval, edema, orthostatic hypotension, weight gain, and extrapyramidal side effects are common.

- *Antipsychotics*: Drugs like risperidone or quetiapine may be needed occasionally to control episodes of aggression in patients with dementias. However, they should not be continued indiscriminately for long as this may increase the risk of stroke.

Survival

Patients may survive for 8–10 years. Some lived up to 25 years. Death usually occurs due to secondary infections, heart disease, or malnutrition.

Vascular Dementia[5]

Onset of cognitive deficits associated with a stroke can occur but often no clear history of stroke may be present but on magnetic resonance imaging (MRI) of brain there may be multiple small, undiagnosed cerebrovascular accidents that could accidentally be found. Abrupt onset of symptoms with stepwise deterioration can occur. Focal findings on neurological examination could be found with or without infarcts on MRI/computed tomography (CT) of brain. These findings often have no clear relationship.

Most patients previously categorized as either Alzheimer's type or vascular type dementias that may probably have components of both types of dementias (mixed dementia). The reason perhaps is that the likelihood of Alzheimer's and vascular disease significantly increases with age, therefore, likelihood of both does as well. Moreover, in a country like India, there is high risk of cardio and vascular illnesses so there is a possibility of dementia being a mixed one. It is noteworthy that vascular risk factors predispose to AD is a new hypothesis and vascular factors are a pathophysiological link between the two. Anticholinesterases, antidepressants, and off and on antipsychotics are the mainstay of treatment. Risk factors like diabetes, hypertension, and coronary artery disease need to be controlled.

Parkinson's Disease Dementia[6]

About one-third of patients with Parkinson's disease (PD) may develop dementia. Risk factors include age over 70 years and depression apart from a diagnosis of PD. Confusion/psychosis or facial masking upon presentation could be presenting features. Recurrent hallucinations and delusions may occur. Those with hallucinations and motor control difficulty have higher risk of dementia. Treatment is done with the help of cholinesterase inhibitors (e.g. rivastigmine). Antipsychotics should be used in very low dose with extreme caution as they may worsen PD. Antidepressants (SSRIs) may be needed. Clonazepam may be given for rapid eye movement (REM) sleep disturbance.

Levodopa may be associated with increased confusion and psychosis.

Dementia with Lewy Bodies[7]

Dementia with Lewy bodies includes 10–20% of all dementias. Compare to PD, Lewy bodies are found in substantia nigra. There may be overlap with AD and PD.

Clinical features include visual hallucinations which appear early in the course of disease, parkinsonism, fluctuating cognition, dysautonomia, sleep disorders, and neuroleptic sensitivity (do not use antipsychotics). Memory changes may appear in the later course of disease. Treatment is same as that of PDD.

Normal Pressure Hydrocephalus[8]

Normal pressure hydrocephalus has a typical triad consisting of:

- Gait disturbance
- Urinary incontinence
- Cognitive dysfunction.

Gait disturbance (magnetic/gait apraxia/frontal *ataxia*) is an early feature and is often most responsive to shunting. Cognitive change includes psychomotor slowing, apathy, decreased attention, and urinary urgency or incontinence can occur. Surgical shunting/external lumber puncture drainage of cerebrospinal fluid is the mainstay of treatment.

Frontotemporal Dementia[9]

Frontotemporal dementia occurs both sporadically and in a familial form inherited as an autosomal dominant. It generally presents in the 6th decade of life. The atrophic process concentrates on the frontal and temporal lobes (hence the name frontotemporal dementia).

Frontotemporal dementia consists of deterioration of personality and cognition associated with prominent frontal and temporal lobe atrophy. This is not common but accounts for up to 20% of dementias.

Treatment involves using SSRIs and/or olanzapine/ quetiapine for addressing hyperactivity or aggressive behavior.

Motor Neuron Disease[10]

Motor neuron diseases are a group of diseases which include progressive degeneration and loss of motor neurons with or without similar lesion of the motor nuclei of the brain. Replacement of lost cells with gliosis can occur. Loss of dexterity, slowed movements, loss of muscle strength, stiffness of limbs, or emotional lability can occur.

Symptom management, nutritional issues, respiratory support, therapies to slow disease progression, and/or palliative care are needed for treatment. Noninvasive ventilatory support or ventilatory-assisted respiration may be needed in due course of time.

Riluzole, an antiglutamate, decreases glutamate release and is given in dose of 100 mg daily. It may decrease need for tracheostomy significantly. Liver functions may need to be monitored. Some patients develop granulocytopenia.

Tricyclic antidepressant and SSRIs may be needed for treatment of underlying depression. Baclofen, tizanidine, or dantrolene, etc. are used as antispastic drugs. Stretching exercises could be done by physiotherapists.

Oral Secretions

Symptoms result from inability to clear oropharyngeal secretions. Common pharmacologic treatments include glycopyrrolate 1–2 mg every 4–6 hours, amitriptyline 25–100 mg at night. Transdermal scopolamine patches can also help. Suction machines can be used in refractory cases.

Emotional Lability

Amitriptyline is commonly used at night to relieve this in dose of 25–100 mg at night.

Spasticity

Common pharmacologic treatments include baclofen 10–40 mg three to four times daily. Dantrolene sodium (dantrium) 25 mg up to four times daily can be used. Tizanidine is an option as well and is used in dose of 12–36 mg three times. Diazepam is used in dose of 2–5 mg three times daily. Botulinum toxin has been tried in refractory cases. Physical and occupational therapy is used regularly.

Associated Symptoms

Dysphagia and respiratory symptom need management.

CONCLUSION[11,12]

Proper history taking, diagnosis and evaluation of a patient of dementia are the mainstay of dementias. Drugs can help a patient of dementia and ease out caregiver burden. Unfortunately, there is no drug to slow down progression but dementia seems preventable. Control of vascular risk factors could potentially prevent dementia. Proper compliance of drugs that have potential to prevent dementia should be ensured. These include antihypertensives, antidiabetics and lipid lowering drugs with or without antiplatelets.

REFERENCES

1. Neurodegenerative Disease Research. (2017). What is neurodegenerative disease? [online] Available from http://www.neurodegenerationresearch.eu/about/what/. [Accessed May, 2018].

2. Alzheimer's Association. (2017). What is dementia? [online] Available from https://www.alz.org/what-is-dementia.asp. [Accessed May, 2018].
3. Alzheimer Society of Canada. (2017). What is dementia? [online] Available from http://www.alzheimer.ca/en/About-dementia/What-is-dementia. [Accessed May, 2018].
4. Robinson L, Tang E, Taylor JP. Dementia: timely diagnosis and early intervention. BMJ. 2015;350:h3029.
5. Kirshner HS. Vascular dementia: a review of recent evidence for prevention and treatment. Curr Neurol Neurosci Rep. 2009;9(6):437-42.
6. Davis CP. (2017). Parkinson disease dementia. [online] Available from https://www.emedicinehealth.com/parkinson_disease_dementia/article_em.htm. [Accessed May, 2018].
7. Tousi B. Diagnosis and management of cognitive and behavioral changes in dementia with Lewy bodies. Curr Treat Options Neurol. 2017;19(11):42.
8. Shprecher D, Schwalb J, Kurlan R. Normal pressure hydrocephalus: Diagnosis and treatment. Curr Neurol Neurosci Rep. 2008;8(5):371-6.
9. Warren JD, Rohrer JD, Rossor MN. Clinical review: Frontotemporal dementia. BMJ. 2013;347:f4827.
10. Orrell RW. Motor neuron disease: systematic reviews of treatment for ALS and SMA. Br Med Bull. 2010;93:145-59.
11. Dhikav V, Singh P, Anand KS. "https://www.ncbi.nlm.nih.gov/pubmed/23731967" Medication adherence survey of drugs useful in prevention of dementia of Alzheimer's type among Indian patients. Int Psychogeriatr. 2013;25(9):1409-13. doi: 10.1017/S1041610213000744. Epub 2013 Jun 4.
12. Dhikav V, Anand KS. "https://www.ncbi.nlm.nih.gov/pubmed/22850312" Are vascular factors linked to the development of hippocampal atrophy in Alzheimer's disease? J Alzheimers Dis. 2012;32(3):711-8. doi: 10.3233/JAD-2012-120928. Review.

CHAPTER

10

Drug Treatment of Stroke

STROKE

Stroke is also called as "brain attack". Stroke is an acute neurological deficit of vascular origin with focal dysfunction and may last for more than 24 hours. Transient ischemic attack or TIA is a neurological deficit of vascular origin lasts from few minutes to hours and resolves within 24 hours.[1] Stroke is one of the leading cause of morbidity and mortality in India. Long-term care and rehabilitation is needed for the survivors.

Speedy diagnosis, rapid access to imaging, quick thrombolysis, and rapid access to supportive therapy are good prognostic factors. Secondary prevention is the key.

Focused history taking and physical examination is a must. One should also assess if there are any contraindications to thrombolytic therapy. Neurologic assessment, e.g. facial paresis, arm drift/weakness, and abnormal speech indicate high positive predictive value for stroke. Measuring vitals, glucose and noncontrast CT.

Head is needed within 3.5 hours of stroke to distinguish intracranial hemorrhage from ischemic stroke.

Rapid surgical/radiological intervention in arterial disease (carotid/vertebral) is fast becoming preferred modality in carefully selected cases. Figures 10.1 and 10.2 give details of the window of intervention.

TYPES OF STROKE

- *Ischemic*: Major strokes are ischemic. Approximately 80% of ischemic strokes are caused by embolism from heart, aortic arch, or extracranial arteries to the brain. Rests of the stroke are called as hemorrhagic.
- *Hemorrhagic*: Traumatic, spontaneous, hypertensive, angiopathy like amyloid angiopathy, aneurysmal rupture, arteriovenous malformation rupture,

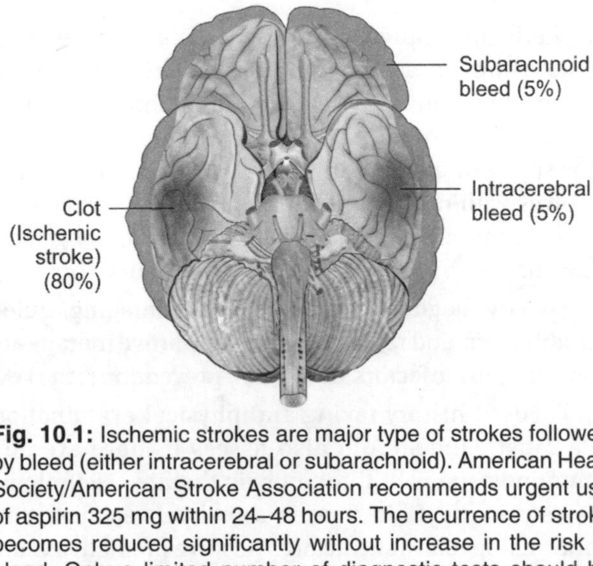

Fig. 10.1: Ischemic strokes are major type of strokes followed by bleed (either intracerebral or subarachnoid). American Heart Society/American Stroke Association recommends urgent use of aspirin 325 mg within 24–48 hours. The recurrence of stroke becomes reduced significantly without increase in the risk of bleed. Only a limited number of diagnostic tests should be performed during acute phase.

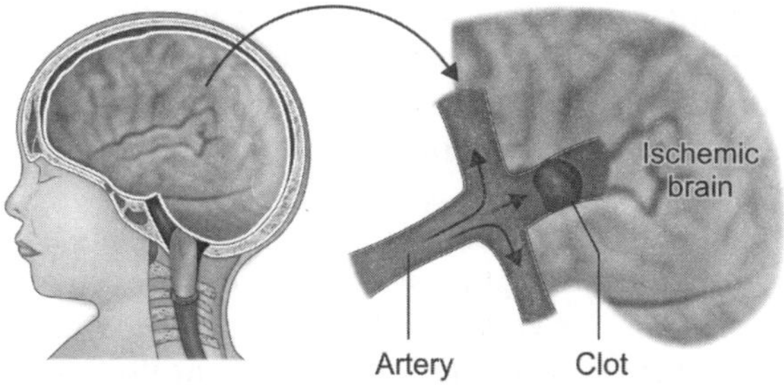

Fig. 10.2: Ischemic strokes represent a window period of 3.5 hours during which the ischemic brain can be salvaged (hence the saying *time is brain*).

TABLE 10.1: Causes of stroke.
• Ischemic stroke (Major types; about 80%)
• Atherosclerotic disease
• Cardioembolic
• Other causes
• Cervical artery dissection
• Endocarditis
• Vasculitis
• Hypercoagulable state
• Herniation
• Hemorrhagic stroke (less common; 20%)
• Intracerebral hemorrhage (ICH)
• Subarachnoid hemorrhage (SAH).

bleeding into tumors or drug abuse like cocaine and amphetamine use, etc. could be the reasons behind. Table 10.1 summarizes causes of stroke.

MANAGEMENT OF STROKE[2,3]

Acute Care

Time of ischemic stroke symptom onset is critical. If unknown, then time the patient was last awake and free of stroke symptoms should be counted as zero time.

When in the emergency room, one would have to assure the optimal perfusion and oxygenation. One of the important things is to protect the cervical spine and secure the airway. Support oxygenation and ventilation may be necessary and one should assure appropriate circulation.

Complete blood counts including platelets count, electrolyte profile, glucose, international normalized ratio (INR), activated partial thromboplastin time (aPTT), serum troponin, and electrocardiogram and X-ray chest gold be done in all cases.

Imaging

A noncontrast head scanning is the initial imaging (first 7 days) study of choice. This is not only readily available but is also very sensitive for blood in the acute phase. However, it should be noted that it is not sensitive for acute ischemic stroke.

Noncontract computed tomography (CT) head may additionally shows signs of ischemia in the first 3 hours. Loss of gray/white matter distinction or hypodensity can be seen. Mass effect, surrounding edema, or hyperdense middle cerebral artery (MCA) sign could be found. One would have to reevaluate the time of symptom onset, if early signs of ischemia are present.

Thrombolysis

Thrombus = clot, lysis = destruction of cells means lysing the clot. Thrombolysis is achieved by using rtPA (alteplase), which is recombinant tissue plasminogen activator. As per American Stroke Association, the only Food and Drug Administration (FDA) approved treatment of acute stroke is tPA.[4]

Plasmin is the enzyme that degrades fibrin, the protein which is the main constituent of blood clots and activates the release of plasmin as plasminogen. It reverses underperfusion, allowing ischemic penumbra to recover. Minor bleeding may occur in about 25% of patients, but about 1% patient may have serious bleed in brain.[5] The following are the contraindications. Box 10.1 details the contraindications of tPA.

Thrombolysis using intravenous tissue plasminogen activator within 3 hours or within 4.5 hours is the standard of care in patients needing immediate thrombolysis. The earlier tPA is administered, the higher the likelihood of a positive neurologic outcome. Endovascular Intra-arterial mechanical thrombectomy is another option. For proximal large vessel occlusion of anterior circulation (intracranial internal carotid, middle cerebral, anterior cerebral, etc.) it should be done within 6 hours of last-seen normal. The same can follow tPA administration also.

Antithrombotic treatment, e.g. aspirin 160 to 325 mg is given within 48 hours. High dose statin, e.g. atorvastatin 80 mg is contnued. Anticoagulation is done only in cardioembolic stroke. Intravenous anticoagulants are not recommended during first 48 hours after acute ischemic stroke but warfarin can be started for small or moderate-sized infarct after 24 hours.

Why thrombolysis?

Thrombolysis reduces the size of ischemic damage (infarct) by restoring blood flow. Cells in the brain,

Box 10.1: Contraindications of tissue plasminogen activator (tPA) in stroke.[5]

- Concomitant head injury
- Active bleeding
- Bleeding ulcers
- Pregnancy
- Recent surgery
- Uncontrolled hypertension.

i.e. neurons die over time. Prompt treatment with a thrombolytic agent (rtPa—alteplase) may promote reperfusion and improve functional outcomes.

When to thrombolyse?

Pharmacologically, rtPA is a recombinant form of tPA and has a short half-life. It is hence given by intravenous (IV) bolus followed by IV infusion.[6]

Thrombolysis must be done within 4.5 hours of stroke and should follow the strict inclusion criteria.[7] rtPA has been licensed for IV use in under 80s years of age. Consultant decision is a must for intra-arterial, 80+ patients. Dramatic increase in poststroke quality of life may occur if the patients have been selected carefully. Treatment of acute stroke is done as per National Institutes of Health (NIH) scores (*see* Box 10.1).

Indications of Thrombolysis

Treatment with rtPA should be started early (within 3 hours) and the intracranial bleeding excluded. Age should be below less than 80 years and early major infarction should be excluded using noncontrast CT (parenchymal hypoattenuation or brain swelling more than one-third of MCA territory). Blood pressure (*BP) should be below less than 185/110 mm Hg and patient should not be on anticoagulants, e.g. warfarin or heparin.* Facilities for close monitoring should be available. Severity categories are given in Table 10.2.

TABLE 10.2: National Institutes of Health (NIH) score categories.

NIH score	*Clinical interpretation*
0–5	Mild
5–15	Moderate
15–20	Severe
>20	Very severe

Main inclusion criteria for thrombolysis is patient presenting within 4.5 hours since onset of symptoms or last known normal. Exclusion criteria include head trauma or stroke in last 3 months, previous intracranial bleed, intracranial tumor, arteriovenous malformation, or aneurysm, recent intracranial or intraspinal surgery, active internal bleeding, bleeding diatheses.

Managing Hypertension

Managing BP aggressively is not recommended. However, following are situations when it should be done (see here). Mostly, the BP reduction should be gradual, except in few situations (Box 10.2).

If the patient is receiving thrombolytic therapy attempt should be to maintain SBP ≤185 mm Hg and DBP ≤110 mm Hg. Afterwards one can stabilize and maintain BP <180/105 mm Hg for at least 24 hours after thrombolytic treatment. In patients receiving no thrombolytic therapy, BP should not be treated acutely unless hypertension is extreme SBP>220 mm Hg or DBP>120 mm Hg or other acute issues exist. When treatment is indicated, cautious lowering of blood pressure by approximately 15% during the first 24 hours should be done.

Nitroglycerin is the agent of choice and can be either given as a patch or an IV drip. One can paste 1–2 inches to skin or as an IV drip; 5 mcg/min, increased later in increments of 5–10 mcg every 3–5 minutes.

Box 10.2: Situations warranting aggressive lowering of blood pressure.

- Hypertensive encephalopathy
- Nephropathy
- Cardiac failure
- Myocardial infarction
- Preeclampsia
- Intracerebral bleed
- Blood pressure more than 200 mm Hg.

Nitroprusside is an alternative drug and is given in dose of 0.3–10 mcg/min/kg as an IV drip with continuous BP monitoring. One would have to check thiocyanate levels in case the patient has been given prolonged infusion. One should avoid nifedipine.

If hypertension is associated with the intracranial bleeding, then it would have to be treated aggressively. One can elevate head of bed and use drugs like labetalol, nitroglycerin, nitroprusside, or furosemide. One should avoid nifedipine and keep systolic less than 160 mm Hg and diastolic less than 100 mm Hg.

Managing Glucose

Since high glucose is associated with worse outcomes after stroke, one should manage either the established concomitant diabetics or acute hyperglycemia at time of infarct. This is because insulin is a neuroprotective.

Fever

Fever is likely to worsen outcome and hence one should treat these patients with paracetamol or ibuprofen, or both.

Seizures

Seizures are an important complication of stroke and occur in 5% of acute strokes. Seizures are usually generalized tonic-clonic. Possible causes include severe strokes, cortical involvement, or past history of seizure disorder.

Benzodiazepines such as lorazepam (1–2 mg IV) or diazepam (5–10 mg IV) is given. One can also give phenytoin 15 mg/kg loading dose, at 25–50 mg/min infusion with cardiac monitor.

Transient Ischemic Attack

Patients who had a suspected TIA are at lower risk of stroke. They should have aspirin (300 mg daily) started immediately. A neurological assessment and investigations had started as soon as possible, but definitely within 1 week of onset of symptoms. The drug should be continued for at least 2 weeks following initial episode following which a definitive treatment can be considered.[8,9] Aspirin can be given with proton pump inhibitor to avoid gastric irritation.

HEMORRHAGIC STROKE[2]

Patient may be unconsciousness or with dysarthria, dysphagia. If the Glasgow Coma Scale score less than 8, intubation should be done. One should avoid hyperventilation or hypoventilation. Nil per orally order should be followed until swallow assessment completed. Begin mobilization as soon as clinically safe. Head end of the bed should be elevated.

The goal is to reduce cerebral edema and maintain cerebral perfusion. Higher BP goals are there with ischemic stroke compared to hemorrhagic stroke. Infarction size and edema increase with acute and chronic hyperglycemia so managing sugar is important. Seizures are common after hemorrhagic stroke and are nonconvulsive associated to with higher National Institutes of Health Scores, a midline shift, and tend to predict poorer outcomes.

PROPHYLAXIS OF STROKE

Usual drugs that patient will have to be given are diuretic, antihypertensive, antiplatelets, or antithrombotics. One will have to address the risk factors include hypertension, TIAs, smoking, previous stroke, diabetes, and arrhythmias, e.g. atrial fibrillation or established carotid artery disease.

It should be kept in mind that majority of strokes are preventable if we are able to manage risk factor such as hypertension, smoking, atrial fibrillation, and improve physical activity. Another important issue is that more than half of the total strokes are related to uncontrolled hypertension, and hence it is by far the most important factor that needs to be controlled.[4]

VENOUS STROKE

Cerebral venous sinus thrombosis needs urgent attention and needs full anticoagulation by maintaining INR between 2 and 3.[9]

CONCLUSION

Stroke is a neurological emergency and "time is brain". After the acute phase is over, long-term management with antihypertensives, antidiabetics (if indicated), lipid lowering, antiplatelets and anticoagulants (if indicated) Addressing risk factors, e.g. Diabetes, hypertension, dyslipidemias can signifcantly affect the prevalance of stroke in a nation like India. Regular exercise, stress reduction/management and early treatment of conditions that can potentially cause stroke (e.g. Arterio-venous malformation) can prevent stroke.

REFERENCES

1. American Heart Association (AHA). (2013). Guidelines for the early management of patients with acute ischemic stroke. [online] Available from https://www.aan.com/Guidelines/home/GetGuidelineContent/581. [Accessed May, 2018].
2. Langhorne P. (2000). Organisation of acute stroke care. [online] Available from https://academic.oup.com/bmb/article-pdf/56/2/436/860427/56-2-436.pdf. [Accessed May, 2018].
3. Williams J. (2016). Acute stroke management and interventions. [online] Available from www.stlouisapn.org/.../acute-stroke-management-and-interventions-2016-apn-confere. [Accessed May, 2018].

4. American Stroke Association. (2017). Stroke treatments. [online] Available from http://www.strokeassociation.org/STROKEORG/AboutStroke/BLS/Stroke-Treatments_UCM_310892_Article.jsp#.WbnTuvMjHDc. [Accessed May, 2018].
5. Florida Hospital. (2017). Side effects of tissue plasminogen activator (tPA). [online] Available from https://www.floridahospital.com/tissue-plasminogen-activator-tpa/side-effects-tissue-plasminogen-activator-tpa. [Accessed May, 2018].
6. Klabunde RE. (2017). Cardiovascular pharmacology concepts: Thrombolytic (fibrinolytic) drugs. [online] Available from http://www.cvpharmacology.com/thrombolytic/thrombolytic. [Accessed May, 2018].
7. Jauch EC. (2017). Acute management of stroke. [online] Available from https://emedicine.medscape.com/article/1159752-overview. [Accessed May, 2018].
8. American Heart Association (AHA). (2016). 2015 AHA/ASA focused update of the 2013 guidelines for the early management of patients with acute ischemic stroke regarding endovascular treatment. [online] Available from https://www.strokeassociation.org/idc/groups/heart-public/@wcm/@hcm/@gwtg/documents/downloadable/ucm_487907.pdf. [Accessed May, 2018].
9. National Institute for Health and Care Excellence (NICE). (2008). Stroke: diagnosis and initial management of acute stroke and transient ischaemic attack (TIA). [online] Available from https://www.nice.org.uk/guidance/cg68/documents/acute-stroke-and-tia-clinical-guideline-nice-version-for-consultation2. [Accessed May, 2018].

CHAPTER

11

Drug Treatment of Neuropathies

What is pain?

Pain is most common sensation brining patient to the doctor. Broadly, pain is an unpleasant sensory and emotional experience associated with actual or potential tissue damage or described in terms of such damage.[1]

It is important to note that the pharmacological treatment of neurologic pain relies on evidence from large randomized controlled trials. A good response to the drug means, at least half of the patients should have an acceptable relief of pain. Causes of neuropathy are given in Figure 11.1.

Neuropathic pain[1] is a neuropsychiatric condition in which pain is initiated or caused by a primary lesion or dysfunction in the nervous system. Understanding the complexity of neuropathic pain becomes the cornerstone for appropriate diagnosis and management. Diabetic neuropathy is very common condition affecting nerves. Flowchart 11.1 gives broad outlines of pathophysiology.

Successful management depends on realistic patient-physician expectations and an individualized,

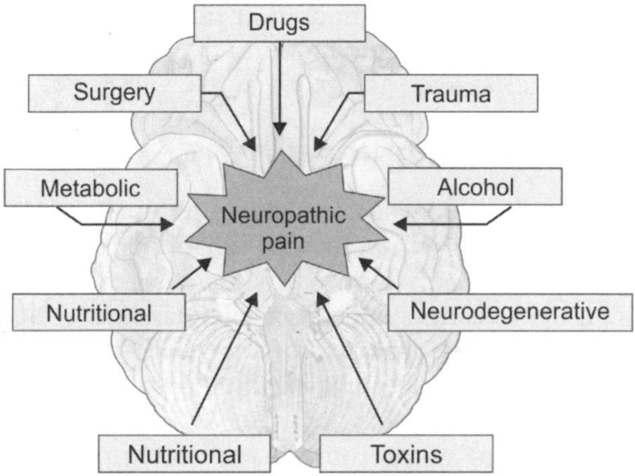

Fig. 11.1: There are several causes of neuropathy pain, e.g. metabolic (e.g. diabetes), trauma, infections, nutritional deficiencies, toxins, drugs, and alcohol, etc. Pharmacological treatment of neuropathic pain relies on evidence from randomized controlled trials in modern medicine. Despite advances in pain research considerable number of patients may not get relief.

Flowchart 11.1: Diabetic neuropathy is the major type of neuropathy and is triggered by increase in blood sugar and propounded by its toxic effects. There are several good treatment options available for painful diabetic neuropathy. Response is defined as a "30–50% reduction in pain severity".

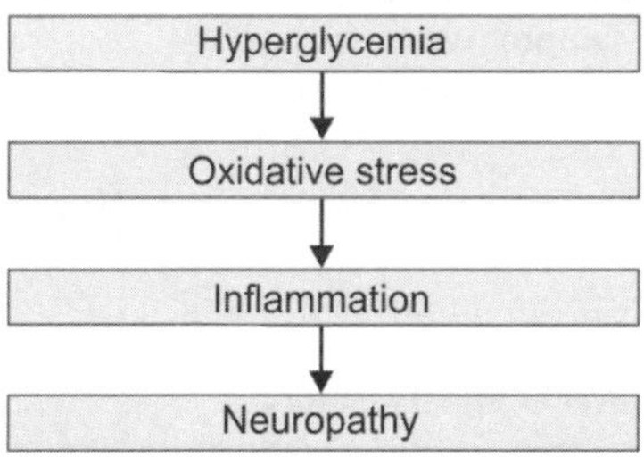

multidisciplinary approach that takes advantage of the ever-evolving armamentarium of evidenced-based treatments.[2,3]

TREATING CHRONIC PAIN[4-6]

The International Association for the Study of Pain (IASP) defines pain as "an unpleasant sensory or emotional experience which we primarily associate with tissue damage or describe in terms of such damage, or both". Neuropathic pain is pain initiated or caused by a primary lesion or dysfunction of the peripheral or central nervous system.

Treatment goals include: balancing efficacy, safety and tolerability, reducing baseline pain, and exacerbations and improving function and quality of life. New agents and new uses for existing agents offer additional treatment options. Neuropathic pain is particularly troublesome and there are several challenges of neuropathic pain (Box 11.1).[7] There are some features, however, that suggest the presence of neuropathic pain (Box 11.2). Common clinical examples of neuropathic

Box 11.1: Challenges posed by neuropathic pain.[7]

- No consensus on definition
- Pain perception is subjective
- Signs and symptoms may change
- Patients not believed about symptoms
- Diagnosis difficult.

Box 11.2: Features of neuropathic pain.

- Lancinating/burning/pricking/stabbing type
- No ongoing tissue damage
- Delay in onset after nerve injury
- Spontaneous paroxysmal electric shock sensation
- Pain with numbness
- Presence of neurologic deficit.

pain are given in Box 11.3. It is important to differentiate acute versus chronic neuropathic pain (Table 11.1). One should differentiate central causes from peripheral causes (Box 11.4).

Box 11.3: Common neuropathic pain syndromes.

- Trigeminal neuralgia
- Postherpetic neuralgia
- Diabetic mononeuropathy
- Entrapment syndrome
- Ischemic neuropathy
- Phantom limb
- *Post-traumatic neuralgia*:
  - *Metabolic*: DM, amyloid
  - *Toxic*: Alcohol, taxanes
  - *Infective*: HIV
  - *Autoimmune*: GBS
  - *Hereditary*: Fabry's disease
  - Malignancy.

(DM: diabetes mellitus; GBS: Guillain-Barré syndrome; HIV: human immunodeficiency virus)

TABLE 11.1: Acute and chronic neuropathic pain.

Characteristics	*Acute*	*Chronic*
Cause	Known	Unknown
Pain duration	Short	Long
Treatment	Short-lived, self-limiting pain; underlying cause needs treatment	Pain control needed; underlying cause may or may not be treatable

Box 11.4: Central causes of pain.

- Spinal cord injury
- Prolapsed disk
- Stroke
- Multiple sclerosis
- Parkinson's disease
- Surgical lesions.

SENSORY SYMPTOMS IN NEUROPATHIC PAIN

Sensations could be impaired. They include numbness, tingling, burning, paresthetic, paroxysmal, lancinating, electric-like, shooting or deep, dull, and bone-like ache.

Signs/Symptoms

Allodynia meaning pain from a stimulus that does not normally evoke pain by stimuli, e.g. thermal or mechanical could be presenting symptom. Hyperalgesia meaning exaggerated response to a normally painful stimulus could also occur.

PATHOPHYSIOLOGY OF CHRONIC PAIN

Chemical excitation of nonnociceptors could be the primary event. Recruitment of nerves outside of site of injury could be followed by excitotoxicity and sodium channels activation. This can lead to ectopic discharge and deafferentation later. Central sensitization could be maintained by peripheral input and could lead to chronic pain. Sympathetic involvement and antidromic neurogenic inflammation could produce protracted painful state. More than one mechanism of action is likely involved. Neuropathic pain may result from abnormal peripheral nerve function and neural processing of impulses due to abnormal neuronal receptor and mediator activity.

GOALS OF TREATING PAIN

There are several goals of treating pain. The first goal is to establish a clear diagnosis of pain. One would have to identify underlying causes of neuropathy. One should identify comorbid conditions and evaluate psychosocial factors as well. The evaluation of the functional status (activity levels) is a must. One would have to develop targeted treatment plan so that one can easily determine when to refer to specialist or multidisciplinary team (pain clinic).

MANAGEMENT OF NEUROPATHIC PAIN

One should note the onset and duration of pain. Also the location/distribution of the pain should be determined. One should note the quality, intensity, aggravating, and relieving factors. A mention should be made of associated features or secondary signs/symptoms. Associated factors could be mood/emotional distress. Also, there could be functional activities impairment as well. Treatment response to earlier treatment should be done.

Nonpharmacological Management

Biofeedback and relaxation therapy have been tried with variable success. Also physical and occupational therapy could be done in selected cases. Cognitive/behavioral strategies need to be chalked out for individual cases. One could suggest approaches such as yoga/meditation/guided imagery as well. However, the controlled trials for the same are lacking. Acupuncture has been tried and transcutaneous electrical nerve stimulation has been used with some success.

Pharmacological Management

Classification

- *Reducing sodium channel activity*:
  - *Na^+ channel blockers*:
    - Phenytoin
    - Lignocaine
    - Oxcarbazepine.

- *Reducing central sensitization:*
  - *N-methyl-D-aspartate (NMDA) receptor antagonist*:
    - Ketamine
    - Amitriptyline
    - Methadone.
  - *Alpha-2 delta blockers*:
    - Gabapentin
    - Pregabalin.
  - *Strengthening local inhibitory controls*:
    - *Gamma-aminobutyric acid (GABA)-B-agonist*: Baclofen.
    - *Opioids*:
      Oxycodone
      Tramadol.
  - *Descending inhibition from brain*:
    - Clonidine
    - Tricyclic antidepressants.

Combination of medications may be needed to manage pain: topicals, anticonvulsants, tricyclic antidepressants, serotonin-norepinephrine reuptake inhibitors, and opioids.

Classes of agents with efficacy demonstrated in multiple, randomized, controlled trials for neuropathic pain are given here in the Box 11.5.

Though there are several options available for the treatment of neuropathic pain, one should always consider safety and tolerability when initiating treatment. The choice depends upon several factors, however, the Box 11.6 gives rough outlines. Details of individual drugs are given here.

Gabapentin

Gabapentin has multimodal action and blocks alpha-2 delta receptors which have a role in pain modulation. The drug reduces ectopic neuronal activity, and decreases central sensitization and reduces glutamate activity.

Box 11.5: Major classes of drugs for neuropathic pain.

- *Topical analgesics*:
  - Capsaicin
  - Lidocaine patch 5%.
- *Anticonvulsants*:
  - Gabapentin
  - Lamotrigine
  - Pregabalin.
- *Antidepressants*:
  - Nortriptyline
  - Desipramine.
- *Opioids*:
  - Oxycodone
  - Tramadol.

Box 11.6: Available choices for neuropathic pain.

- *Carbamazepine/oxcarbazepine/lamotrigine*:
  - Trigeminal neuralgia.
- *Duloxetine*:
  - Painful diabetic neuropathy.
- *Gabapentin*:
  - Postherpetic neuralgia.
- *Lidocaine patch 5%*:
  - Postherpetic neuralgia.
- *Pregabalin*:
  - Peripheral diabetic neuropathy
  - Postherpetic neuralgia.
- *Postherpetic neuralgia*:
  - Gabapentin/pregabalin.
- *Diabetic neuropathy*:
  - Carbamazepine
  - Phenytoin
  - Gabapentin
  - Lamotrigine
  - Pregabalin.
- *Human immunodeficiency virus (HIV)-associated neuropathy*:
  - Lamotrigine.
- *Central poststroke pain*:
  - Lamotrigine
  - Gabapentin.

The drug is given in dose of 300–3,000 mg/daily. Common side effects include dizziness, sedation, weight gain, etc. Contraindication includes hypersensitivity reaction. Gabapentin is a Food and Drug Administration (FDA) approved drug for postherpetic neuralgia. As an anticonvulsant, it has uncertain mechanism. The drug has limited intestinal absorption. It is usually well tolerated; serious adverse effects are rare. Dizziness and sedation can occur. There are no clinically significant drug interactions. Peak time to achieve plasma concentration is 2–3 hours after oral absorption and the drug has an elimination half-life of 5–7 hours. Usual dosage range for neuropathic pain is up to 3,600 mg/day given in three to four times daily doses.

Pregabalin

Pregabalin has similar mechanism to that of gabapentin. The drug is used in dose of 75–600 mg/day in divided doses. Common side effects include dizziness, sedation, confusion, peripheral edema, weight gain, etc. Contraindication is hypersensitivity reaction.

Antidepressants

Antidepressants are very popular for neuropathic pain. They have multiple mechanisms of action. Randomized controlled trials and meta-analyses demonstrate benefit of tricyclic antidepressants (especially amitriptyline, nortriptyline, and desipramine) for postherpetic neuralgia and diabetic neuropathic pain. Onset of analgesia, however, is variable. Analgesic effects independent of antidepressant activity, however, the improvement in depression may be noted as well. Improvements in insomnia, anxiety may occur concomitantly. Desipramine and nortriptyline have fewer adverse effects. Amitriptyline is tolerated poorly by elderly. Commonly reported adverse effects (generally anticholinergic) are given here in the Box 11.7.

Safety of antidepressants in neuropathic pain: Desipramine and nortriptyline are likely to have lesser side effects compared to imipramine and doxepin have comparatively more side effects.

Amitriptyline

Amitriptyline is used in dose of 10–75 mg/day and side effects are mainly anticholinergic, constipation, and confusion, etc. Common contraindications include narrow angle glaucoma, urinary retention, and second or third-degree heart block.

Desipramine

Desipramine is given in dose of 100–200 mg daily and can be increased to 300 mg daily. The dose should be gradually increased. Elderly patients need much lower dose, e.g. 25–100 mg daily.

Nortriptyline

The drug is used in dose of 25 mg three to four times daily in maximum dose of 150 mg daily. The drug is monitored in plasma (50–150 ng/mL).

Box 11.7: Common side effects of antidepressants.

- Blurred vision
- Cognitive changes (e.g. memory lapses)
- Constipation
- Dry mouth
- Orthostatic hypotension
- Sedation
- Sexual dysfunction
- Tachycardia
- Urinary retention.

Imipramine

Imipramine is used in dose of 25–100 mg daily. The dose can be increased to 300 mg/daily. The drug should be started in low dose and can be slowly increased.

Doxepin

Doxepin is started in dose of 75 mg orally once daily and it can be increased to 150 mg daily.

Ketamine

Ketamine, an NMDA antagonist is given in dose of 0.25 mg/kg–1,000 mg/day. Side effects include delirium, hallucinations, confusion, night mares, etc. Contraindications include hypersensitivity and psychiatric disorders.

Tramadol

Tramadol is used in dose of 50 mg twice daily to 400 mg/daily. Side effects include sedation and nausea. Precautions are needed in elderly where side effects could be more.

Opioids

Opioids are centrally acting powerful analgesics and opioids can be effective in neuropathic pain. Since, tolerance, addiction, and dependence could be issues in chronic neuropathic pain, they should be titrated for therapeutic efficacy. Fixed-dose regimens generally preferred over as per needed regimens. One should document treatment plan and anticipate outcomes. Most opioid adverse effects could be controlled with appropriate specific management (e.g. prophylactic bowel regimen, use of stimulants).

Tolerance, addiction, and dependence: Physical dependence means withdrawal syndrome arises if drug discontinued, dose substantially reduced, or antagonist (e.g. naloxone, naltrexone) administered. Tolerance means greater amount of drug needed to maintain therapeutic effect, or loss of effect over time.

Pseudoaddiction means behavior suggestive of addiction, and it may be caused by undertreatment of pain.

Addiction (psychological dependence) is a psychiatric disorder characterized by continued compulsive use of substance despite harm.

TOPICAL TREATMENT

Lidocaine 5% in pliable patch and up to three patches applied once daily directly over painful site. The drug can be used for 12 hours on and 12 hours off basis. Recently published data indicate safety and efficacy of randomized controlled trials on postherpetic neuralgia. Drug interactions and systemic side effects unlikely and most common side effect is application-site sensitivity. Clinically insignificant serum lidocaine levels appear to be of no consequence upon topical administration. Mechanical barrier decreases allodynia. Lidocaine is used in dose of 5 mg/kg over 1 hour. Side effects include hypotension, neurotoxicity, and sedation.

INTERVENTIONAL TREATMENT

A number of interventional treatments have been tried.

- Neural blockade involves sympathetic blocks for chronic regional pain syndrome (CRPS-I and II; called respectively as reflex sympathetic dystrophy and causalgia).
- Neurolytic techniques such as alcohol or phenol neurolysis have been used with pulse radiofrequency.

- Stimulatory techniques such as spinal cord stimulation and peripheral nerve stimulation have been used.
- Medication pumps fitted with fentanyl or baclofen are used commonly in intrathecal area. The pump is designed to release the drug slowly.

RECENT ADVANCES[8]

Botulinum toxin has been tried for low back pain. Lidocaine patch 5% has also been tried for low back pain, osteoarthritis, diabetic, and human immunodeficiency virus (HIV)-related neuropathy, with gabapentin. Oxycodone has been tried in diabetic neuropathy. Gabapentin has been found to be useful in HIV-related neuropathy, diabetic peripheral neuropathy, and others. Levetiracetam has been found to be useful for neuropathic pain and migraine. Oxcarbazepine has been tried in neuropathic pain related to diabetic neuropathy. Bupropion and fentanyl (transdermal) are being evaluated for low back pain.

Pharmacoresistance

Pharmacoresistance occurs when even rotation of drugs fail to produce response or produces intolerable side effects. Patients may have lowers quality of life, increase in intensity of symptoms despite using expensive medications. A neuropathic pain condition is resistant to pharmacotherapy when mono or a rational combination treatment using drugs proved efficacious in randomized trials fail in providing pain relief after an appropriate duration of treatment with adequate dosage.

CONCLUSION

In the future, ability to determine the relationship between the pathophysiology and symptoms/signs may help target therapy. Newer targets are being searched for addressing the components of chronic pain.

REFERENCES

1. National Institute for Health and Care Excellence (NICE). (2013). Neuropathic pain in adults: pharmacological management in nonspecialist settings. [online] Available from https://www.nice.org.uk/guidance/cg173. [Accessed May, 2018].
2. Neuropathic Pain. (2017). Neuropathy and neuropathic pain: an overview. [online] Available from https://www.emedicinehealth.com/neuropathic_pain_nerve_pain/article_em.htm. [Accessed May, 2018].
3. Markman J, Narasimhan SK. (2014). Neuropathic pain. [online] Available from https://www.merckmanuals.com/professional/neurologic-disorders/pain/neuropathic-pain. [Accessed May, 2018].
4. Webberley H. (2017). What is peripheral neuropathy? [online] Available from https://www.medicalnewstoday.com/articles/147963.php. [Accessed May, 2018].
5. National Health Trust Choices. (2017). Peripheral neuropathy treatments. [online] Available from https://www.nhs.uk/conditions/peripheral-neuropathy/treatment/. [Accessed May, 2018].
6. Drugs.com. (2016). Doxepin dosage. [online] Available from https://www.drugs.com/dosage/doxepin.html. [Accessed May, 2018].
7. Drugs.com. (2016). Nortriptyline dosage. [online] Available from https://www.drugs.com/dosage/nortriptyline.html. [Accessed May, 2018].
8. American Chronic Pain Association. (2017). Neuropathic pain. [online] Available from https://www.theacpa.org/conditions-treatments/conditions-a-z/neuropathic-pain/. [Accessed May, 2018].

CHAPTER

12

Drug Treatment of Demyelinating Diseases

WHAT IS MULTIPLE SCLEROSIS?

Multiple sclerosis (MS) is a chronic, progressive, and degenerative disorder of the central nervous system (CNS) characterized by disseminated demyelination of nerve fibers of the brain and spinal cord.[1]

EPIDEMIOLOGY

Multiple sclerosis usually affects young to middle-aged adults, with onset between 15 years and 50 years of age. Women affected more than men. The disease has unknown cause, probably related to infectious, immunologic, and genetic factors. Possible precipitating factors include infection, physical injury, emotional stress, excessive fatigue, pregnancy, poor general health, etc.[2]

PATHOPHYSIOLOGY

Myelin sheath is basically a segmented lamination that wraps axons of many nerve cells. It increases velocity of nerve impulse conduction in the axons as to facilitate neuronal conduction. Myelin sheath is composed of myelin, a substance with high lipid content. In MS, chronic inflammation, demyelination, and gliosis (scarring) of CNS nerves occur. The disease is initially triggered by a virus in genetically susceptible individuals. Subsequent antigen-antibody reaction leads to demyelination of axons (Figs. 12.1A and B).

Patient may complain of noticeable impairment of function and by the time it happens, a significant number of nerves may have been affected. Myelin can luckily regenerate, and symptoms disappear, resulting in a remission. Myelin can be replaced by glial scar tissue and without myelin, nerve impulses slow down. With destruction of axons, impulses are totally blocked results in permanent loss of nerve function.

TYPES OF MULTIPLE SCLEROSIS[3]

- *Relapsing-remitting multiple sclerosis (RRMS)*:
  - Characterized by periods of flare-ups and remission
  - Accounts for 85% of MS patients.
- *Primary progressive multiple sclerosis (PPMS)*:
  - Slow continuous worsening of disease from onset
  - Only about 10%.
- *Secondary progressive multiple sclerosis (SPMS)*:
  - Initial period of relapsing-remitting, then steady worsening of disease
  - 50% of patients diagnosed with RRMS develop into this variety within 10 years without drug treatment.
- *Progressive relapsing multiple sclerosis (PRMS)*:
  - Steady worsening with acute relapses
  - Different from RRMS in that disease progresses during relapses
  - Only about 5%.

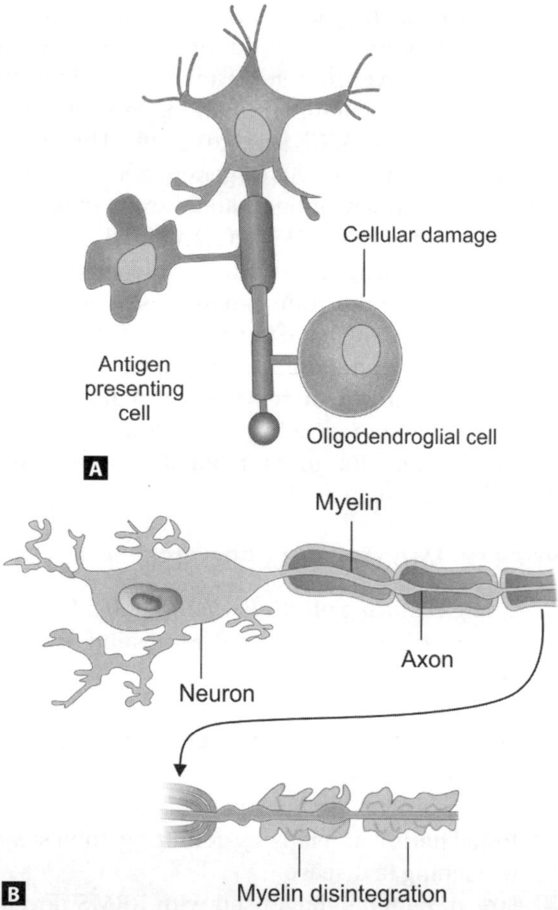

Figs. 12.1A and B: Multiple sclerosis involves inflammation in the central nervous system (CNS) where the demyelinating lesions called plaques develop and become indurated (therefore, the hardening is called as sclerosis). The disease process consists of loss of myelin, disappearance of oligodendrocytes, and proliferation of astrocytes. Changes result in plaque formation with plaques scattered throughout the CNS. Initially the myelin sheaths of the neurons in the brain and spinal cord are attacked, but the nerve fiber is not affected.

CLINICAL FEATURES[4]

In the beginning, vague symptoms occur intermittently over months and years. MS may not be diagnosed until long after the onset of the first symptom. The disease is characterized by chronic, progressive deterioration in some patients and remissions and exacerbations in others. Common signs and symptoms include motor, sensory, cerebellar, and emotional problems. Cognitive change is a significant late presenting feature. The following domains are affected:

- *Motor manifestations*: Weakness or paralysis of limbs, trunk, and head could occur leading to diplopia (double vision), scanning speech, and spasticity of muscles can occur.
- *Sensory manifestations*: Numbness and tingling are common. Some patients could have blurred vision, vertigo and tinnitus, and decreased hearing and chronic neuropathic pain.
- *Cerebellar manifestations*: Nystagmus is not uncommon. Ataxia and dysarthria can occur. Lack of coordination in articulating speech may be evident. Dysphagia may be late feature.
- *Bowel and bladder functions*: This is one of the most disabling manifestations. Constipation and spastic bladder could occur. Small capacity for urine results in incontinence of urine. Flaccid bladder large capacity for urine and no sensation to urinate.
- *Sexual dysfunction*: This is particularly troublesome in young patients and manifestation as erectile dysfunction in men and decreased libido in both sexes. Difficulty with orgasmic response, painful intercourse, and decreased lubrication may be other presenting features.

DIAGNOSING MULTIPLE SCLEROSIS

Diagnosis is based primarily on history and clinical manifestations. The key is ruling out other causes of symptoms as there is no single definitive diagnostic test. Magnetic resonance imaging (MRI) demonstrates presence of plaques and the basis of diagnosis should be primarily the history, clinical manifestations, and presence of multiple lesions over time measured by MRI. Certain laboratory tests are used as adjuncts to clinical examination.

TREATMENT

Drug Therapy[3-5]

Drug therapy is the cornerstone of treatment of MS (Box 12.1). The aims of treating patient of MS are threefold: (1) treating acute relapse, (2) symptomatic management, and (3) disease modification.

Glatiramer

Glatiramer is used to reduce frequency of relapse in remitting and relapsing form of MS. The drug works by modifying immune response. The recommended dose is 20/mg daily given subcutaneously.

Alemtuzumab

Alemtuzumab is a recombinant monoclonal antibody that binds to CD52 (a type of lymphocyte antigen). This

Box 12.1: Available options in multiple sclerosis.

- Interferons beta
- Ocrelizumab
- Dimethyl fumarate
- Fingolimod
- Natalizumab
- Teriflunomide
- Alemtuzumab.

initiates antibody-dependent cell lysis. The drug is used for relapsing form of MS. Due to serious adverse effects, the drug is used in refractory form of MS.

Fingolimod

This is the first of the oral treatments approved for treating MS. The drug can reduce clinical exacerbations and disability. The work perhaps works by reducing lymphocyte migration to the brain. The dose is 0.5 mg given once daily.

Natalizumab

This is used as a monotherapy to delay the physical disability and reduce exacerbations. Progressive leukoencephalopathy is a side effect. Progressive multifocal leukoencephalopathy, a rare brain infection may lead to death or severe disability. Once develops, only supportive treatment is available. Immunosuppressive drugs along with natalizumab are not given and is given as a monotherapy. This infection can occur in patients who have used it for 2 years or longer or those infected with John Cunningham Virus (JCV).

The most common side effects of netalizumab are headache, urinary tract and pulmonary infection, lung infections, pain in limbs, vaginitis, stomach-area pain, joint pain, depression, diarrhea, rash, nose and throat infections, and nausea, etc.

The drug is given in dose of 300 mg IV infusion over one hour every month.

Teriflunomide

Teriflunomide is another oral immunomodulatory drug that with anti-inflammatory effects. The drug works by inhibiting dihydroorotate dehydrogenase, a mitochondrial enzyme involved in pyrimidine synthesis. It is indicated for relapsing forms of MS.

Teriflunomide is used for the treatment of relapsing forms of multiple sclerosis in the dose of 7 mg or 14 mg (orally) on daily basis.

Disease-modifying Drugs

- *ABC treatments*: ABC refers to the three major brand names of this category of drugs: (1) Avonex, (2) Betaseron/Betaferon, and (3) Copaxone.
- *Chemotherapeutic agents*: Mitoxantrone is most commonly employed for the same. The drug is available as 2 mg/mL injection and is given as 12 mg/mL as a short intravenous infusion every 3 months.
- *Corticosteroids*: Most popular drug treatments for modifying course of disease are corticosteroids. They work by regulating aspects of the immune system. Methylprednisolone 1 g everyday for 3–5 days is usual way in which patients are treated during acute exacerbations. High dose prednisolone (1,200 mg) has also been used safely. Redness of face, increased appetite, weight gain, gastrointestinal upset, mood swings, and fluid retention can occur as side effects.
- *Symptomatic treatment*:[6] Wide variety from antidepressants (depression) to laxatives (bowel dysfunction) to anticonvulsants (pain/altered sensations).
- *Interferon beta-1a*: Interferon beta-1a is used for RRMS and SPMS with relapses. The drug is produced by recombinant deoxyribonucleic acid (DNA) technology using genetically engineered Chinese Hamster Ovary cells into which the human interferon beta gene has been introduced. The resulting amino acid sequence is identical to human interferon beta. Interferon beta-1b was the first drug approved in MS for relapsing form of MS to reduce exacerbation. The drug has good efficacy in first clinical episode of MS.

Mechanisms by which it exerts its effects not fully understood. Pharmacokinetics of the drugs in MS patients has not been evaluated. Recommended dosage of 30 μg is injected intramuscularly once weekly. Not recommended subcutaneously—adverse reactions mainly at site of injection. The drug does not have any interactions with other drugs. Safety of doses above 60 mcg has not been evaluated.

Corticosteroids

Corticosteroids treat acute exacerbations by reducing edema and inflammation at the site of demyelination. Corticosteroids do not affect the ultimate outcome or degree of residual neurologic impairment from exacerbation.

Immunosuppressive Therapy[7-9]

Multiple sclerosis is considered an autoimmune disease; the potential benefits of immunosuppressive therapy should be counterbalanced against potentially serious side effects.

Antispasmotics (Muscle Relaxants)

Baclofen is most commonly used drug for reducing spasticity of MS. The drug not only relieves muscle spasm but may also increase performance. It can be given orally or as an intrathecal pump. Tizanidine, an alpha-2 agonist is another drug used for the same purpose.

Physical Therapy

Physiotherapy relieves spasticity and increases coordination. So, one can train the patient to substitute unaffected muscles for impaired ones.

Nutrition

Nutritional therapy includes megavitamins and diets consisting of low-fat, gluten-free food, and raw vegetables. High-protein diet with supplementary vitamins is often prescribed.

INDIAN ACADEMY OF NEUROLOGY GUIDELINES OF MULTIPLE SCLEROSIS[10]

- *Education*: Acute relapse may be triggered by infections and it needs to be treated aggressively. Patients can be vaccinated. Patients need to be educated about physical trauma and stressful life events.
- *Steroids*: It is important to know that not all relapses need treatment. Steroids are indicated for disabling replaces such as optic neuritis, motor impairment, ataxia, etc. Steroids promote apoptosis of T cells and have potent anti-inflammatory effects. The drug is given in dose of 1 g/daily for 3–5 days. Generally such a course is limited to three courses per year. One should exclude urinary tract infections before starting the drug.
- *Interferon beta*: A weekly dose of 30 mg (interferon beta-1a) is given intramuscularly (Avonex) or alternatively, Rebif, another brand is given as a dose of 22 mg or 44 mg weekly up to three times. One should begin with lower dose.
- *Mitoxantrone*: The drug is given in remitting-relapsing or SPMS. Patient needs to be monitored for cardiotoxicity.
- *Natalizumab*: The drug is given as a monthly infusion and patient needs to be watched out for progressive multifocal leukoencephalopathy.

MULTIPLE SCLEROSIS IN PREGNANCY

Relapse rates are low in pregnancy. Disease-modifying drugs should be stopped prior to conception (at least 3 months). The drugs can be started once the breastfeeding is over. Interferons and natalizumab are category C drugs while mitoxantrone is a category D drug.

CONCLUSION

Multiple sclerosis is an demyelinating disease of inflammatory origin affecting central nervous system. The disease may result in a wide range of neurological symptoms and accumulating disability over the years. Continuing education is the key in enabling the person to actively participate in their management of disease. There are about one dozen disease modifying therapies available with varying degree of efficacy for treatment of multiple sclerosis. They mainly reduce the risk of relapse and preserve neurological functions. Their adverse effects, long-term toxicities should be taken into account while prescribing them on long-term basis.

Corticosteroids, interferon-beta, mitoxantrone, natalizumab, fingolimod, teriflunomide, dimethyl fumarate, alemtuzumab, rituximab, are nowadays commonly used.

REFERENCES

1. Luzzio C. (2018). Multiple sclerosis treatment and management. [online] Available from https://emedicine.medscape.com/article/1146199-treatment. [Accessed May, 2018].
2. National Health Trust Choices. (2017). Multiple sclerosis: treatment. [online] Available from https://www.nhs.uk/conditions/multiple-sclerosis/treatment/. [Accessed May, 2018].

3. National Multiple Sclerosis Society. (2017). Treating multiple sclerosis. [online] Available from https://www.nationalmssociety.org/Treating-MS. [Accessed May, 2018].
4. Multiple Sclerosis. (2017). Types and treatment of multiple sclerosis. [online] Available from https://www.multiplesclerosis.com/us/treatment.php. [Accessed May, 2018].
5. Multiple Sclerosis Society (2017). Treatment and therapies in multiple sclerosis. [online] Available from https://www.mssociety.org.uk/what-is-ms/treatments-and-therapies. [Accessed May, 2018].
6. Anderson L. (2018). Multiple sclerosis: What's new in MS treatment options? [online] Available from https://www.drugs.com/slideshow/multiple-sclerosis-1054. [Accessed May, 2018].
7. Medscape. (2017). Mitoxantrone dosing and side effects. [online] Available from https://reference.medscape.com/drug/mitoxantrone-342186. [Accessed May, 2018].
8. MedBroadcast. (2017). Facts about multiple sclerosis. [online] Available from http://www.medbroadcast.com/condition/getcondition/multiple-sclerosis. [Accessed May, 2018].
9. Costello K, Harris CJ. (2006). An overview of multiple sclerosis: diagnosis and management strategies. [online] Available from https://www.medscape.com/viewarticle/527706_7. [Accessed May, 2018].
10. Pandit L, Murthy JM. Treatment of multiple sclerosis. Ann Indian Acad Neurol. 2011;14(Suppl 1):S65-9.

CHAPTER

13

Drug Treatment of Traumatic Head Injury/Spinal Cord Injury

INTRODUCTION

Head trauma[1] is the leading cause of death in people under the age of 30 years. Males have 2–3 × frequency of brain injury than females. Head trauma in India occurs mostly due mainly to motor vehicle accidents and assaults. Road crossers and pedestrians are at greatest risk followed by bikers and cyclist.

More than 200,000 people in the world live with the disability caused by head injures alone.

TYPES OF HEAD INJURY[2]

Primary

Head injury of this type can lead to injury to scalp, skull fracture, or surface contusion/laceration. Serious injuries can lead to intracranial hematoma or diffuse axonal injury, diffuse vascular injury.

Secondary

Hypoxia-ischemia, swelling/edema, and raised intracranial pressure associated with head injury can be the reasons behind secondary head injury. Meningitis/brain abscess may occur.

DIAGNOSIS

Computed tomography (CT) is the minimal brain imaging investigation required for patients with minor head injury and any one of the following:

- *High risk (for neurological intervention)*:
  - Glasgow Coma Scale (GCS) score less than 15 at 2 hours after injury.
  - Suspected open or depressed skull fracture.
  - Any sign of basal skull fracture [hemotympanum, *raccoon* eyes, and cerebrospinal fluid (CSF) otorrhea].
  - Vomiting more than or equal to two episodes.
  - Age more than or equal to 65 years.
- Sensitivity of these rules (100%), specificity (69%), and CT ordering proportion (32%).

Computed tomography without contrast is the modality of choice in acute trauma (fast, available, and sensitive to acute subarachnoid hemorrhage and skull fractures). Magnetic resonance imaging (MRI) is useful in nonacute head trauma (higher sensitivity than CT for cortical contusions, diffuse axonal injury, and posterior fossa abnormalities).

OPEN AND CLOSED HEAD INJURIES

Closed Head Injury

Closed head injury often results from falls, motor vehicle crashes, etc. Focal damage and diffuse damage to axons can occur. Effects of head injury tend to be broad or diffuse. Importantly, there is no penetration to the skull in the closed form of head injury.

Open Head Injury

This often results from road traffic accidents in India and bullet wounds, etc. in the Western world. The result is largely focal damage. Penetration of the skull occurs and effects can be serious.

EFFECTS OF HEAD INJURY

Tissue damage, internal bleeding in the brain, and swelling occurs leading to loss of consciousness, seizures, delirium, etc. Post-traumatic amnesia is a dreaded sequel of head injury.

Epidural Hematoma

- Epidural hematoma is the collection of blood and clot between dura mater and bones of the skull. The source is the middle meningeal artery tear of bleeding from dural venous sinuses.
- Clinical features include brief loss of consciousness, headache, drowsiness, dizzy, nausea, vomiting, and rapid clinical deterioration (typically *talk and die*).

Subdural Hematoma

Subdural hematomas (SDHs) result most frequently from tearing of a bridging vein between the cerebral cortex and a draining venous sinus. These are of three types:

1. Acute occurring within less than 24 hours.
2. Subacute occurring between 24 hours and 2 weeks.
3. Chronic after 2 weeks.

Intracerebral Hematoma

Intracerebral hematoma is formed within brain tissue and caused by shearing or tensile forces that mechanically stretch and tear deep small caliber arterioles. Most common in temporal and frontal regions. Clinical features depend on site involved.

Concussion

Concussion is temporary and brief interruption of neurological function after minor head injury due to shearing/stretching of white matter fibers at the time of impact or temporary neuronal dysfunction. Patients may complain of headache, confusion, and amnesia. CT/MRI cannot detect this.

ASSESSING HEAD INJURY

One would have start with determining the severity of head injury. The hints can be provided by the duration of loss of consciousness, initial score on GSC, length of post-traumatic amnesia, etc. (Table 13.1).

MANAGEMENT

History and initial clinical assessment is important. One should do primary and secondary survey. Primary survey is done with an intent of airway maintenance with cervical

TABLE 13.1: Determining clinical severity of head injury.

Loss of consciousness time	*Glasgow Coma Scale score*	*Severity of head injury*
0–20 minutes	13–15	Mild
20 minutes to 6 hours	9–12	Moderate
>6 hours	3–8	Severe

spine protection. Secondary survey includes thorough history taking if there is an accompanying person present. One should do examination head to toes and apply GCS. Detailed neurological examination is needed.

Breathing and ventilation is the utmost priority and one can premedicate with lidocaine, 1 mg/kg intravenous (IV) 2 minutes prior to attempting intubation.

One should maintain mean arterial pressure more than 90 mm Hg adequate. Hematocrit should be more than 30%. Also, check for Cushing reflex.

One should do imaging studies only after the spine has been stabilized fully.

- *Primary treatment*: The treatment starts with head end elevation (30°) and IV fluids (e.g. normal saline). One should maintain normovolemia. Hypotonic/ glucose containing fluids should not be used. Serum sodium levels are monitored daily.
- *Mannitol*: Mannitol, an osmotic diuretic is given in doses up to 1 g/kg. It decreases intracranial pressure and maintains cerebral blood flow, cerebral perfusion pressure, and brain metabolism. The aim should be to decrease intracranial pressure within 6 hours. The drug also expands volume and improves oxygen (O_2) carrying capacity of the blood. It has diuretic effect so the net intravascular volume is reduced.
- *Furosemide*: This is a powerful diuretic. The drug is given to reduce intracranial tension in conjunction with mannitol. The drug is used in dose of 0.3–0.5 mg/kg. It should not be used in hypovolemia.
- *Hyperventilation*: It has *no role as prophylaxis in 24 hours where the focus is on hemodynamic stability. Later, when patient stabilizes one can use this to reduce* partial pressure of carbon dioxide in arterial blood ($PaCO_2$) which can cause cerebral vasoconstriction. This is to maintain $PaCO_2$ of 25–35 mm Hg. This may be the last resort for reducing intracranial pressure.

- *Barbiturates*: Barbiturates are effective in reducing intracranial pressures in refractory to other measures. The drug (e.g. phenobarbitone) is not used in presence of hypotension/hypovolemia.
- *Anticonvulsants*: Phenytoin is used in the loading dose of 18–20 mg/kg and maintenance dose of 100 mg every 8 hourly.
- *Surgical treatment*: Depending upon the individual cases, scalp wounds cleaning and debridement may be needed. Elevation of depressed fractures will be needed. Craniotomy and evacuation of hematoma may be urgently needed. Cranial decompression for reduction of intracranial pressure may be needed.

RECOVERY

Recovery following head injury is a multistage process. This may continue for days or even months or years sometimes. The timescale differs for each person. Seizures, amnesia, or neurological deficits could be consequences. The major long-term deficits are given in Box 13.1.

Cognition

- Attention
- Concentration
- Memory
- Speed of processing
- Confusion

Box 13.1: Major areas affected.

- Cognitive
- Sensory loss
- Seizures
- Social-emotional
- Neurological deficits.

- Perseveration
- Impulsiveness
- Language processing
- *Executive functions.*

Sensory

- Vision
- Hearing
- Smell
- Vestibular
- Taste
- Touch
- Balance.

Pain

Chronic pain.

Bowel and Bladder

Control of bowel and bladder.

Sleep Disorders

- Loss of stamina
- Appetite changes
- Regulation of body temperature
- Menstrual difficulties.

Types

- Subarachnoid hemorrhage (SAH)
- Subdural hematoma
- Epidural hematoma
- Subdural hygroma
- Intraventricular hemorrhage.

SPINAL CORD INJURY

Injury to spinal cord is not common but is often serious. Incidence of the problem is 10–12,000/year in developed world. In a nation like India, it is likely to be more. Most patients are young males and about 20% are females. About half of cases have complete section of cord and cervical area is quite vulnerable. Due to serious nature of this problem, about half of the victims die.

Primary Injury

Initial insult to cord, local deformation of the cord, and vertebrae are significant factors in injury. Energy transformation plays a key role.

Secondary Injury

Biochemical cascade after the injury is important here. Cellular processes lead to compounding of injury. *Most acute therapies aim to limit secondary injury cascade.* Free radicals and apoptosis play important roles in secondary injury to cord.

Clinical Features

Spinal Shock

Transient flaccid paralysis is the usual outcome of moderate to severe spinal cord injury. Areflexia follows.

Neurogenic Shock

This is the next thing to come; loss of sympathetic tone, vasomotor, and cardiac regulation. Hypotension with relative bradycardia occurs.

Types of Spinal Cord Injuries

Complete

Absence of sensory and motor function in lowest sacral segment after resolution of spinal shock.

Incomplete

Presence of sensory and motor function in lowest sacral segment (indicates preserved function below the defined neurological level).

Classification

American Spinal Injury Association (ASIA) divides spinal cord injury into five types:

1. A = Complete—no sacral motor/sensory
2. B = Incomplete—sacral sensory sparing
3. C = Incomplete—motor sparing (<3)
4. D = Incomplete—motor sparing (>3)
5. E = Normal motor and sensory.

Management[3]

- Attempt should be done to stabilize spine and maintain proper breathing.
- During spinal shock, the blood pressure should be maintained and kept above 90 mm Hg.
- Oxygenation and perfusion of the injury cord should be maintained. Attempt should be made to use mechanical ventilation, if needed.
- Maintain sinus rhythm and treat any cardiac arrhythmia. Atropine may be needed for bradycardia.
- Urine output should be maintained (30 mL/h) and Foley's catheter should be put in place.
- Inotropic support with dopamine and dobutamine may be needed. Low dose dopamine 2–5 µg/kg/min IV may be given.

- Hypothermia should be prevented.
- High dose prednisolone is helpful in reducing motor and sensory deficits if given within 8 hours of injury. The drug is given in dose of 30 mg/kg.

CONCLUSION

Most head injuries are mild cases. Cases of head injury with mild to moderate injury make good recovery; and residual deformities are uncommon. However, severe injury with Glasgow coma scale score <8, presence of focal neurological signs, signs of increased intracranial pressure or signs of basal skull fracture may have grim prognosis. The initial aim of management of a patient with a serious head injury is prevention of secondary brain damage. Both systemic and neurological complications can occur. Likewise spinal cord injury may involve any part of the cord or the tail end (Cauda equina). Permanent changes in motor power, sensory system or bowel and bladder can occur. Prompt diagnosis and treatment are the keys.

REFERENCES

1. Olson DA. (2016). Head injury treatment and management. [online] Available from https://emedicine.medscape.com/article/1163653-treatment. [Accessed May, 2018].
2. American Association of Neurological Surgeons. (2017). Guidelines for the management of severe traumatic brain injury. [online] Available from https://icnapedia.org/guidelines/secured/1.ppt. [Accessed May, 2018].
3. Chin LS. (2017). Spinal cord injuries treatment and management. [online] Available from https://emedicine.medscape.com/article/793582-treatment#d10. [Accessed May, 2018].

CHAPTER

14

Drug Treatment of Cervical Spondylosis, Low Backache

CERVICAL SPONDYLOSIS

Cervical spondylosis[1] is a disorder caused by abnormal strains on cervical vertebrae with or without degeneration and mineral deposits in the attachments of the cervical vertebrae. The disorder results in pain and weakness in the neck and arm, and changes in sensation. Neck pain is a common complaint and tends to occur with increasing frequency after the age of 30 years. So basically, cervical spondylosis, is an age-related process that affects many components of the cervical spinal column. It is important to know that most episodes of neck pain are short-lived and tend to respond to nonoperative management.

Clinical Spectrum

The spectrum of cervical spondylosis ranges from axial neck pain to radiculopathy to frank myelopathy. Physical examination findings correlated with diagnostic imaging studies that can aid in diagnostic evaluation. Almost all patients with symptomatic cervical degenerative disease without neurologic involvement can be managed nonoperatively. Surgery for patients with myelopathy is a reasonable option to prevent disease progression.

General Features[1]

The clinical manifestations of neck disorders range from midline posterior neck pain to the neurologic sequelae of cervical nerve root or spinal cord compression. Axial neck pain may radiate from the base of the skull down to the upper trapezius region. Cervical radiculopathy involves compression of a nerve root, with pain radiating down the arm in an anatomic distribution. Cervical myelopathy is characterized by dysfunction of the spinal cord. This may be caused by cord compression, vascular abnormalities, or a combination of both.

Pathophysiology[1,2]

Degeneration of the intervertebral disk can lead to pain referred to the neck, posterior skull, and/or upper shoulders.[1] This may occur as a natural consequence of the normal aging process with a resulting decrease in the water content of the disk. Disk degeneration can be affected by many external factors including repetitive occupational mechanical strain and a history of diving or heavy weight lifting.

Acute herniation of the disk material posteriorly may result in impingement of the nerve root and/or spinal cord resulting in pain. The distribution of pain in cervical radiculopathy often fits a dermatomal distribution characteristic for each particular nerve root. When cord compression occurs, the changes within the cord can be caused by acute compression by the disk material, as well as compression of the vascular supply to the cord.

Cervical spondylosis may involve loss of disk space height. As a result of the degeneration within the disk and the decreased intervertebral height, altered spinal biomechanics ensure with osteophytes forming along the area of the disk space as well as posteriorly along the facet joints. This can be associated with nerve root and spinal cord compression.

- *Signs and symptoms*: Neck pain is perceived by the patients from an existing primarily within the axial portion of the spine. Pain may radiate to the base of the skull or to the midupper periscapular region. The pain may involve the posterior trapezius muscles or the posterior deltoids. The pain itself may be limited to a focal area or may involve a more global region. Night pain is common because the neck becomes a weight-bearing area and muscles are relaxed.
- *Physical examination*: When there is severe neck spasm, the head may be flexed laterally to that side or even rotated. Examination should include inspection of the symmetry of the paraspinal muscles as well as the trapezius and shoulder musculature. Any signs of atrophy must be noted. Strength and range of motion of the shoulder should be tested, as well as examination for focal tenderness within the shoulder (to help rule out the shoulder as a source of potential pain or to define coexistent shoulder disease).

CERVICAL RADICULOPATHY

- *Signs and symptoms*: Cervical radiculopathy implies pain traveling on the basis of an anatomic distribution to the shoulder or down the arm. Patients describe sharp pain and tingling or burning sensations in the involved area. There may be sensory or motor loss corresponding to the involved nerve root, and reflex activity may be diminished.
- *Physical examination*: The shoulder abduction relief sign is characterized by having the patients place

the palm of his hand flat onto the top of his skull; this causes symptomatic relief of the radicular pain. Spurling's test is performed by having the patient extend the neck and rotate and laterally bend the head toward the affected side; an axial compressive force is then applied to the top of the patient' head. The test is positive when the maneuver reproduces the patients typical radicular arm pain.

- *Pathophysiology*: Herniation or degeneration of an intervertebral disk may produce specific radicular patterns, depending on the level of involvement. C5–6 and C6–7 are far more commonly involved than C7–T1 or C4–5. Pain radiates to the shoulder or lateral arm and dorsal forearm. Anesthesia and paresthesias may be present in the thumb and index finger. Weakness, involves the biceps and wrist extensors. The brachioradialis or biceps reflex is often decreased or absent (C6–7 nerve root). The pain distribution is similar to that of a C7 radiculopathy. Anesthesia and paresthesias involve the index and middle fingers. Weakness is noted in the triceps, wrist flexors, and finger extensors. The triceps reflex may be reduced (C7–T1 nerve root affected). Pain may occur along the medial aspect of the upper arm and forearm. Anesthesia and paresthesias involve the ring and small fingers. Weakness, if present, is noted in the finger flexors and intrinsic musculature of the hand. The triceps reflex may be reduced.
- *Signs and symptoms*: Cervical myelopathy alone in the absence of radiculopathy is painless. This is due to the fact that there is spinal cord compression only. The pain becomes apparent only when compression of the spinal cord is accompanied by compression of the nerve root (myeloradiculopathy).

Symptoms associated with spinal cord compression include gait disturbances with balance difficulty, fine motor dysfunction in the hands, and motor weakness. Bowel and bladder dysfunction is found late in the progression of cervical myelopathy.

- *Physical examination*: Hoffmann's reflex is often present, which is elicited by flicking the middle finger of the patient and observing forced finger and thumb interphalangeal joint flexion. There can be up going toes (e.g. positive Babinski's reflex) as well as associated clonus at the ankles. Myelopathy-related hand abnormalities include atrophy of the thenar musculature and an inability to maintain the ring and small fingers is an extended and adducted position (e.g. finger escape sign). Lhermitte's sign involves flexion of the neck with an electric shock-like sensation extending down the axial spine and/or extremities.

CERVICAL MYELOPATHY

- *Physical examination*: Lower extremity strength needs to be tested including hip flexors, knee extensors and flexors, hip abductors and adductors, ankle dorsiflexors, and plantar flexors, etc. Function of the extensor hallucis longus and peroneals should be tested as well. Sensory examination should include light touch, pinprick, and vibration sense using a tuning fork. Reflex examination should include the triceps, biceps and brachioradialis, quadriceps, and the Achilles tendon. Another abnormal finding is the inverted radial reflex, characterized by spontaneous finger flexion when the examiner attempts to elicit a brachioradialis reflex. Gait should be tested during normal walk as well as with toe to heel walking.
- *Diagnosis*: Laboratory studies should include routine blood workup, a complete blood count with

differential, and an erythrocyte sedimentation rate (ESR) and C-reactive protein (CRP). These results will most commonly be abnormal when an infectious or malignant process is involved. An electrophysiology study may be helpful in defining a specific level when nerve compression is present. Such a study may also be helpful in ruling out other neurologic disorders including peripheral neuropathy.

A plain X-ray with anterior/posterior, lateral, and oblique views could show lot of important findings. Degeneration can often be noted within the disk spaces and the facet joints. There are often osteophytes noted along the area of the disk space and foraminal narrowing can be noted on oblique views. Clinical correlation with patient symptoms is often poor in those older than 40 years.

Myelography can be used to help evaluate nerve root compression as well as compression of the spinal cord. Root compression is manifested by an extradural filling defect with obliteration of the nerve root sleeve. Flattening of the spinal cord can be appreciated on the lateral view. In cases of severe compression, there will be complete obstruction of flow of the myelogram dye. In most clinical situations, this test has given way to the magnetic resonance imaging (MRI).

Computed tomography (CT) is helpful in evaluating the degree of foraminal stenosis caused by bony osteophytes. In combination with myelography, it provides superior imaging compared to myelography alone. Diagnostic features are given in Box 14.1.

- *Differential diagnoses*: Diagnoses one should consider with cervical disk disease are numerous (Box 14.2). Diagnostic guidelines are given here in

Box 14.1: Clinical features of cervical spondylitis.

- Neck pain (may radiate to the arms or shoulder)
- Loss of sensation or abnormal sensations of the shoulders, arms, or legs
- Weakness of the arms or legs
- Neck stiffness that progressively worsens
- Loss of balance
- Headaches, particularly in the back of the head
- Loss of control of the bladder or bowels.

Box 14.2: Differential diagnosis.

- Trauma
- Cervical sprain
- Brachial plexus injury
- Fracture dislocation
- *Inflammatory conditions*: Rheumatoid arthritis and ankylosing spondylitis
- *Infectious*: Diskitis, osteomyelitis
- Soft tissue abscess
- Tumors
- Pancoast' tumor
- Shoulder disorders including rotator cuff disease.

Box 14.3 and common complications are given in Box 14.4.

Imaging

A spine or neck X-ray may show abnormalities that indicate cervical spondylosis, e.g. arthritic changes. A CT scan or spine MRI may be done to confirm the diagnosis. A myelogram may be done to clearly identify the extent of injury. An EMG may also be recommended to know the functional status of nerve muscle junction. An X-ray of the lower (lumbar) spine may reveal degenerative changes in this region.

Box 14.3: Diagnosing spondylitis—points to consider.

- *Age*: The most cases are over 40 years old and men more than women
- Pain in the neck, headache (back of head), shoulder, or radiating pain in the arm or fingers
- Numbness or tingling in the arm or fingers or thumb
- Dizziness
- Loss of balance
- Dry eyes, visual disturbances (e.g. blurred vision, diplopia)
- Tinnitus
- Disturbed concentration and memory
- Hot flash (rarely)
- X-ray, MRI, and CT will find particular problem.

(CT: computed tomography; MRI: magnetic resonance imaging)

Box 14.4: Common complications of spondylitis.

- Chronic neck pain
- Progressive loss of muscle function or feeling
- Permanent disability (occasional)
- Inability to retain feces (fecal incontinence) or urine (urinary incontinence).

Treatment

- *Primary treatment*: Patients with neck pain, with or without radicular symptoms. Lifestyle modifications should be instituted to avoid activities that tend to create or aggravate neck and arm symptoms.[3] A typical activities to modify include athletic activities, sitting at a desk with neck flexion (e.g. reading and typing) for extended periods of time, and driving. An ergonomic assessment of the modern computerized offices often helpful in decreasing day-long stresses to the neck. A soft cervical collar can be used to limit motion and allow the spasm to settle down. The use of two or three pillows at night, in order to decrease reflux symptoms or breathing problems, exacerbate cervical spine problems and should be avoided. Therefore, use of a cervical pillow under the nape of the neck at night helps decrease spasms and pain, as it tends to optimize the position of the neck during sleep. Other modalities such as moist hate and light massage may prove beneficial. Practice guidelines recommend *ACE approach* to neck pain (A = analgesia, awareness, C = counseling, and E = exercises).[3,4]

- *Drugs*: Use of medications including anti-inflammatory medications help decrease the amount of inflammation and provide pain relief. In cases of severe pain, mild narcotics may be useful. Muscle relaxants may also help decrease the amount of spasm and allow or more comfortable periods of rest. Short courses of steroids are sometimes needed to control the inflammatory process. Nonsteroidal anti-inflammatory drugs (NSAIDs) like paracetamol, ibuprofen, and diclofenac sodium are first-line drugs as per practice guidelines.[3,4] Table 14.1 gives details of commonly used drugs. Details of nondrug therapies are given here:
  - *Physiotherapy*: Physical therapy is often useful in the treatment of neck and radicular arm pain, once the phase of severe pain and radicular problems resolve. Modalities including traction, ultrasound, or diathermy can give pain relief. Once the patient's symptoms have begun to decrease, an exercise regimen can be added taking note that this does not exacerbate the neck or arm pain symptoms. Active exercises along with some isometric exercises can help regain the strength of the neck. Clinical practice gudelines[3] indicate that coexisting back pain, poor quality of life, and age over 40 years could be aggravating factors. Exercises to improve coordination,

TABLE 14.1: Various medical treatment options for cervical spondylitis.

Nonsteroidal anti-inflammatory drugs (NSAIDs)	*Corticosteroids*	*Alpha-2 delta blockers*	*Antidepressants*	*Opioids*	*Muscle relaxants*
Ibuprofen is used in dose of 400–800 mg twice or thrice daily and a maximum of 3,200 mg can be used	Oral prednisolone can be used in high dose for short period to relieve inflammation associated with cervical spondylosis	Radicular pain can be reduced by gabapentin	Drugs like amitriptyline reduce pain and produce good deal of sedation to ensure good sleep. Drug can be started in dose of 10 mg night time to 100 mg daily	Used for debilitating back pain unresponsive to other therapies; used in low dose for short duration. Oxycodone, fentanyl, and methadone are used for this purpose	Used extensively in combination with NSAIDs; baclofen, chlorzoxazone, carisoprodol, and tizanidine, are commonly used

strengthening, and enduring exercises may be recommended for these.[3]

- *Surgery*: This is indicated in cases of significant radicular pain that has failed to respond to conservative treatment, or in the presence of significant neurologic deficits. Only a small percentage of patients with cervical spine problems eventually require surgery. However, if considered necessary, the surgical procedure is either an anterior cervical diskectomy and fusion or a posterior laminoforaminotomy. For cases of myelopathy with significant disability, surgery can be a reasonable alternative. The goal of surgery with myelopathy is to prevent progression of the disease. Postoperatively, some patients show improvement from their preoperative neurologic status. For myelopathy, surgery consists of either multiple anterior cervical diskectomies/corporotomies and fusion versus posterior procedures such as laminectomy alone, laminoplasty, or laminectomy and fusion. A small percentage of patients with significant multilevel disease or poor bone quality are good candidates for a combined anterior/posterior procedure. Surgery should be done emergently in the setting of an epidural abscess.
- *Prognosis*: Prognosis for patients with axial neck pain is, in general, good. Surgery for axial neck pain by itself is rarely indicated, except perhaps in the setting of instability. The prognosis for patients with cervical radiculopathy is also, in general, favorable. A significant number of patients tend to respond to nonoperative measures and show significant improvement in 2–3 months after the onset of symptoms. The prognosis for improvement with surgery is

generally favorable. Most patients experience significant improvement in their radicular pain.

Cervical Myelopathy

Cervical myelopathy with early myelopathy and no significant neurologic deficits can initially be followed in an outpatient setting. It should, however, be noted that a high percentage of these patients may slowly deteriorate over time.

The deterioration is often slow and occurs over years; a small percent of cases may display signs and symptoms of rapid progression. In patients with gross findings of myelopathy with significant cord compression and impairment, surgery is a reasonable option. The goal of surgery is to prevent deterioration and promote improvement in their overall neurologic status.

BACK PAIN

Back pain is the second most common cause of missed work days. It is leading cause of disability between ages of 19–45 years. It is number one cause of impairment and occupational injuries. It is important to know that most episodes of low back pain are self-limited.

Episodes of low back pain become more frequent with age. Low back pain is usually due to repeated stress on the lumbar spine over many years (*degeneration*), although an acute injury may cause the initiation of pain. It is important to know that majority of the adults experience back pain at some point in their life. A handful of back pain becomes chronic and males and females are equally affected. One should always ascertain that if it is systemic disease or the cause? Also one needs to know if there is social or psychological distress that prolongs or amplifies symptoms or not. One should also note if there is associated neurologic compromise that requires surgical intervention, e.g. cancer, compression fractures, spinal stenosis, aortic aneurysms, etc.

Osteoporotic fractures without trauma can also occur. Spinal stenosis secondary to degenerative processes and spondylolisthesis is more common. Early radiography recommended and plain radiography limited to patients with findings suggestive of systemic disease, trauma, and failure to improve after 4–6 weeks. CT and MRI are more sensitive for cancer and infections—also reveal herniation and stenosis.

Straight Leg Raising Test

The straight leg raise test is positive if pain in the sciatic distribution is reproduced between 30° and 70° passive flexion of the straight leg. Dorsiflexion of the foot exacerbates the pain.

- *Nerve root pain*: Nerve root pains are often associated with radiculopathy which may present as sciatica. The patients may have herniated disk, foraminal or spinal stenosis, ligamentous hypertrophy, other space filling lesions: cysts, tumor, abscess, etc. Patients may also have viral or immune inflammation.
- *Spinal stenosis*: This is presented by neurogenic claudication (pseudoclaudication) in one or both legs. Radiation to buttocks, thighs, and lower legs can occur. Pain increase with extension (standing, walking) and pain may decrease with flexion (sitting, stooping forward).

Medical Management

Moderate bed rest is useful, however, prolonged bed rest should be avoided. Spinal manipulation and physical therapy may offer help. Medications such as NSAIDs, muscle relaxants are commonly used. For severe back pain, rarely narcotics are used. Aspirin, paracetamol, ibuprofen, diclofenac, aceclofenac, and naproxen are commonly used NSAIDs for low back pain. Ketorolac, tramadol, and diclofenac are available as parenteral medications. Locally applied gels and sprays are very popular in India for low back pain.

Surgical Treatment

Lumbar fusion or replacement with artificial disk may be recommended. "Microdiskectomy" which includes less than half of an inch incision may be used. Patient can go home the same or next day. Good results in up to 90% of cases may be obtained. Residual pain may last up to 6 months postoperatively in others. Results are worse if pain was present for over 8 months before the operation (permanent nerve damage).

Surgery is indicated for low back pain that has been going on for at least 2 years, incapacitating, resistant to physical therapy and medication, and has positive MRI findings (degenerative changes) at L4–5 and/or L5–S1. Surgery may be ineffective unless there is evidence of sciatica, pseudoclaudication, and spondylolisthesis. If no evidence of the conditions mentioned earlier, then cauda equina or progressive neurologic deficit should be existing. A month of nonsurgically trial may be given. Epidural steroids are helpful in some cases. If severe pain or neurodeficits persist, then there is no need to wait and one should do urgent CT/MRI and consider for surgery.

Spinal Stenosis

Conservative management may be useful but for severe persistent pain, decompressive laminectomy may be done. Surgery is better done for pain relief and functional recovery. Intensive exercises help but may be hard to maintain. Antidepressant therapy is useful if patient is depressed but long-term opioids therapy is not recommended. Massage therapy may be helpful. One should referral to pain center if no relief and the therapeutic goal is to optimize daily function. Herniated disks without neurologic deficits may be subjected to diskectomy. Microdiskectomy is nowadays popular and may offer pain relief similar to standard procedure. Laser diskectomy is less effective. Arthroscopic diskectomy appears promising.

Practice Guidelines for Low Back Pain[5]

- *Nondrug treatment*: Nonpharmacological treatment, e.g. heating pad, massage, acupuncture, or manipulation of spine can be used for initial treatment.
- *Drugs*: Nonsteroidal anti-inflammatory drugs or muscle relaxants are used.
- *Chronic back pain*: Interventions such as yoga, or meditation, or muscular relaxation can be used. Biofeedback or cognitive behavioral therapy has been found to be useful.
- *Failure of nondrug therapy*: Drugs such as tramadol, or duloxetine can be used. Do not use opioids in general. They are used only in exceptional cases. If drugs fail, surgery is an option.

CONCLUSION

Musculoskeletal pains include bone pains, which are usually deep, penetrating, or dull. Trauma is usual etiology. One would have to rule out fracture or tumor as the cause of pain. Muscle pain is usually less intense than bone pain, but it can still be quite debilitating. Muscle pain can be caused by an injury, autoimmune reaction, loss of blood flow to the muscle, infection, or a tumor. The pain can also include muscle spasms and cramps, which are far more common. Tendon and ligament pain (e.g. sprains) are usually post-traumatic. This type of musculoskeletal pain often becomes worse when the affected area is stretched or moved. Fibromyalgia may cause pain in the muscles, tendons, or ligaments or all of them together with multiple tender points. The pain is usually in multiple locations and can be difficult to describe. Fibromyalgia is usually accompanied by other symptoms, e.g. anxiety, depression, sleep disturbances, etc.

Joint pains are common and usually produce a stiff, aching, "arthritic" pain. The pain may range from mild to severe and worsens when moving the joint. The joints may also swell. "Tunnel" syndromes refers to musculoskeletal disorders that cause pain due to nerve compression. The disorders include carpal tunnel syndrome, cubital tunnel syndrome, and tarsal tunnel syndrome, etc. The pain tends to spread along the path supplied by the nerve and may feel like burning. These disorders are often caused by overuse, e.g. typing. Diabetes and hypothyroidism are common accompaniments of carpal-tunnel syndrome.

Attempt should be done to know the extent of symptoms, interference in activities of daily living and comfort should always be provided. A detailed diagnostic work up may be needed. Co-existing psychiatric morbidity may need urgent attention too. At times, psychiatric diseases, e.g. anxiety/depression, etc. may present with prominent musculoskeletal complaints.

REFERENCES

1. Isaac Z. (2017). Treatment of neck pain. [online] Available from https://www.uptodate.com/contents/treatment-of-neck-pain. [Accessed May, 2018].

2. WebMd. (2017). Neck pain treatment: overview. [online] Available from https://www.webmd.com/a-to-z-guides/tc/neck-pain-treatment-overview. [Accessed May, 2018].
3. Physiopedia. (2017). Neck pain: Clinical practice guidelines. [online] Available from https://www.physio-pedia.com/Neck_Pain:_Clinical_Practice_Guidelines. [Accessed May, 2018].
4. Teichtahl AJ, McColl G. (2013). An approach to neck pain for the family physician. [online] Available from https://www.racgp.org.au/afp/2013/november/neck-pain/. [Accessed May, 2018].
5. National Institute for Health and Care Excellence. (2017). Low back pain. [online] Available from https://www.nice.org.uk/guidance/conditions-and-diseases/musculoskeletal-conditions/low-back-pain. [Accessed May, 2018].

CHAPTER

15

Drug Treatment of Central Nervous System Infections

INTRODUCTION

Central nervous system (CNS) infections are often life-threatening problems with high associated mortality and morbidity. The presentation may be acute, subacute, or chronic. Clinical findings are an interplay of anatomic site/s of involvement, infecting pathogens, and host response. Vulnerability of CNS to effects of inflammation and edema mandates prompt diagnosis with appropriate therapy if consequences to be minimized.[1]

Some of the infections are given following in Box 15.1.[2]

PATHOGENESIS[3]

Three common bacteria causing brain infections are: (1) *Haemophilus influenzae type b* (Hib), (2) *Neisseria meningitidis*, and (3) *Streptococcus pneumonia*. Vulnerable groups for meningitis include neonates, elderly, and immunosuppressed, etc.

Routes of entry could be hematogenous or neighboring focus, etc. The anatomic defect, e.g. congenital, traumatic,

Box 15.1: Common central nervous system (CNS) bacterial infections.[2]

- Bacterial meningitis
- Meningoencephalitis
- Brain abscess
- Subdural empyema
- Epidural abscess
- Septic venous sinus
- Thrombophlebitis.

or surgical can play important roles. Intraneural pathways could be important as well.

THERAPEUTIC AIMS IN ACUTE CENTRAL NERVOUS SYSTEM INFECTIONS[3,4]

One should promptly recognize the patient with an acute CNS infection syndrome and treat accordingly. Also, one has to rapidly initiate appropriate empiric therapy. In addition, attempts should be made to specifically identify the etiologic agent and adjust the therapies as indicated on prompt basis. One should optimize management of complicating features as well.

CLINICAL ASSESSMENT

Acute cases present within 24 hours while subacute within 7 days. Meningitis becomes chronic if it takes more than 4 weeks. History and physical examination can give useful clues to the cause. Box 15.2 gives details of clinical features of meningitis.

DIAGNOSIS

Cerebrospinal Fluid

One should note down color/clarity/cell counts/white blood cell (WBC) count, chemistries (protein, glucose),

Box 15.2: Clinical features of meningitis.

- Fever
- Headache
- Nuchal rigidity
- Altered mental status
- Photophobia
- Nonspecific symptoms/signs
- Focal neurological signs
- Seizures
- Specific clinical stigmata according to etiological agent
- Children/elderly.

stains (e.g. Gram positive or negative), cultures (routine), and antigen screens, etc. *Streptococcus pneumoniae, Neisseria meningitidis,* and Hib could be positive in 50–100% of patients. Cryptoantigen screen detects *Cryptococcus neoformans,* and is positive in 90–95% of patients with cryptomeningitis. Low glucose could be due to higher bacterial load and suggests bacterial meningitis.

Every patient with meningitis should have cerebrospinal fluid (CSF) obtained unless the procedure is contraindicated. Chemistry and cytologic findings highly suggestive of bacterial meningitis include a CSF glucose concentration below 45 mg/dL, a protein concentration above 500 mg/dL, and a WBC count above 1,000/mm^3. A Gram stain should also be obtained and could be positive in up to 10% of patients. The following features are suggestive of dementia.

Opening pressure more than 180 mm H_2O and WBCs 10–10,000/L. It is important to that in infective bacterial meningitis, neutrophils predominate. Red blood cells are absent in nontraumatic tap. Glucose levels below 40 mg/dL and CSF proteins more than 45 mg/dL are indicative of bacterial meningitis. Gram stains may be positive in more than 60% and CSF culture in more than 80%.

Latex agglutination may be positive in patients with meningitis due to *Streptococcus pneumoniae*, *Neisseria meningitidis*, Hib, *Escherichia coli*, and group B streptococci. Limulus test may be positive in cases of Gram-negative meningitis. Polymerase chain reaction can detect bacterial deoxyribonucleic acid (DNA).

Lumbar Puncture

This is the single most important diagnostic test. It is a mandatory test, especially, if bacterial meningitis is suspected. If lumbar puncture is contraindicated (Box 15.3), one should obtain bacteria count and then begin empirical treatment. CSF features are summarized in Table 15.1.

Imaging

It is usually an overemployed diagnostic modality in the diagnosis of CNS infections. However, it leads to unnecessary delays in treatment and added costs. It is important to know that imaging *per se* is rarely indicated in patients with suspected acute meningitis. This is, however, mandatory in patients with possible focal infection. Increased sensitivity with contrast enhancement could be expected.

Box 15.3: Contraindications of lumbar puncture.

- *Absolute:*
  - Skin infection over site
  - Papilledema
  - Focal neurological signs.
- *Relative:*
  - Increased intracranial pressure (ICP) without papilledema
  - Suspicion of mass lesion
  - Spinal cord tumor
  - Spinal epidural abscess
  - Bleeding diathesis or ↓ platelets.

TABLE 15.1: Cerebrospinal fluid (CSF) features of bacterial meningitis.

Cerebrospinal fluid parameters	*Typical findings*
Opening pressure	200–500 mm H_2O
White blood cell count	1,000–5,000/mm^3 (range = 100–10,000)
Percentage of neutrophils	≥80%
Protein	100–500 mg/dL
Glucose	≤40 mg/dL
CSF-to-serum glucose ratio	≤0.4
Gram stain	Positive in 60–90%
Culture	Positive in 70–85%
Polymerase chain reaction	Useful to detect bacteria

Box 15.4: Penetration of antibiotics inside blood–brain barrier.

- Penicillins
- Cephalosporins
- Chloramphenicol
- Rifampin
- Trimethoprim-sulfamethoxazole combination.

TREATMENT

The chosen antimicrobial must have good activity on the suspected pathogen(s) and should preferably be bactericidal. Adequate CSF diffusion is a good indicator of its potential efficacy and the drug should have acceptable risk of toxicity. The penetrations of antibiotics are given in Box 15.4.

Antibacterial Therapy

Bactericidal therapy is generally necessary to cure meningitis. Bacteriostatic drugs, such as clindamycin and tetracycline, may be inadequate for meningitis.

Chloramphenicol is a bacteriostatic drug for most enteric Gram-negative rods; however, it is usually bactericidal for *Haemophilus influenzae*, *Neisseria meningitidis*, and *Streptococcus pneumoniae* and has been extensively and successfully used to treat meningitis caused by these organisms.

Empirical Therapy

Selected third-generation cephalosporins such as cefotaxime and ceftriaxone have emerged as the beta-lactams of choice in the empiric treatment of meningitis. These drugs have potent activity against the major pathogens of bacterial meningitis with the notable exception of *Listeria*. Ceftazidime, another third-generation cephalosporin, is much less active against penicillin-resistant pneumococci than cefotaxime and ceftriaxone. Ceftriaxone 2 grams given intravenously (IV) very 12 hourly or cefotaxime 2 grams IV every 4–6 hourly plus vancomycin 15 mg/kg every 6–12 hourly can be used. If the patient is more than 50 years, one can also add ampicillin 2 grams IV every 4 hourly (for *Listeria*).

Streptococcus pneumoniae

The conventional approach to the treatment of pneumococcal meningitis was the administration of penicillin alone for 2 weeks in a dose of four million units IV every 4 hours. Good results have also been obtained with third-generation cephalosporins. However, the problem of treating pneumococcal meningitis has recently been compounded by the widespread and increasingly common reports of pneumococcal strains resistant to penicillin. Cefotaxime or ceftriaxone can be used if the minimal inhibitory concentration (MIC) for these drugs is less than 0.5 μg/mL. It is recommended that vancomycin (2 g/day) should be given with cefotaxime or ceftriaxone in the initial treatment of pneumococcal meningitis if there has been beta-lactam resistance noted locally.

Vancomycin should be continued if there is high level penicillin resistance and an MIC more than 0.5 μg/mL to third-generation cephalosporins. If corticosteroids are given, rifampin should be added as a third agent since it increases the efficacy of the other two drugs. The usual duration of therapy is 2 weeks.

Treatment is done using high doses of penicillin, e.g. 1.2 grams (2 million units) given 2 hourly. Please note that some strains have reduced susceptibility to penicillin and some are resistant. Polyvalent vaccines for risk groups, e.g. before splenectomy is available.

Haemophilus influenzae

Haemophilus is a Gram-negative coccobacillus, capsulated strains (type b used predominate). Peak incidence occurs in 2 years old (range = 3 months to 5 years). Incidence has declined greatly since the successful introduction of Hib vaccine. Condition has insidious onset, no rash, and has lower mortality. Treatment is done using cefotaxime or ceftriaxone.

A third-generation cephalosporin is the drug of choice for *Haemophilus influenzae* meningitis. Patients with *Haemophilus influenzae* meningitis should be treated for 5–7 days. For adults, a dose of 2 grams every 6 hours of cefotaxime and 2 grams every 12 hours of ceftriaxone is more than adequate therapy. Pharyngeal colonization persists after curative therapy and may require a short course of rifampin if there are other children in the household who are at risk for invasive *Haemophilus* infection. The recommended dose is 20 mg/kg/day (to a maximum of 600 mg/day) for 4 days.

Neisseria meningitidis

This infection is best treated with penicillin although there are scattered case reports of *Neisseria meningitidis* resistant to penicillin, such strains are still very rare. A third-generation cephalosporin is an effective alternative to penicillin for meningococcal meningitis. A 5 days duration of therapy is usually considered adequate. When penicillin is used, there may still be pharyngeal colonization with the infecting strain which may take some more time for eradication or need alternative therapies. As a result, the index patient may need to take rifampin, a fluoroquinolone, or a cephalosporin.

If meningococcal meningitis confirmed then a change to high doses of benzylpenicillin can be considered. Close contacts in home, school/university, and nursery should be given antibiotic prophylaxis. Rifampicin 600 mg once daily for 2 days or ciprofloxacin 1,000 mg once daily is used. Hospital contacts only need prophylaxis if contact with secretions, e.g. mouth to mouth resuscitation.

Listeria monocytogenes

Listeria has been traditionally treated with ampicillin and gentamicin, as resistance to these drugs is quite rare. Ampicillin is given in typical meningitis doses (2 grams IV every 4–6 hours in adults) and gentamicin is used for synergy. An alternative in penicillin-allergic patients is trimethoprim-sulfamethoxazole (dose of 10/50 mg/kg/day in two or three divided doses). The usual duration of therapy is at least 3 weeks.

Enteric Gram-negative Rods

Prior to the availability of third-generation cephalosporins, it was often necessary to instill an aminoglycoside antibiotic such as gentamicin directly into the cerebral ventricles or given intrathecally. It is now possible to cure these infections with high doses of third-generation antibiotics. A repeat CSF sample should be obtained for culture 2–4 days into therapy to help assess the efficacy of treatment. The duration of therapy should be at least 3 weeks. Meningococcal vaccines are active against many strains of *Neisseria meningitidis*. However, the majority of meningococcal infections are caused by type b Meningococcus for which there is no vaccine. Vaccines for other types (for example type a) are recommended for travelers and to countries with epidemic meningitis. Immunization against meningococci is not warranted as postexposure prophylaxis.

Steroids

The use of steroids as anti-inflammatory agents has been attempted as an adjuvant in the treatment of meningitis. Early administration of corticosteroids such as dexamethasone for pediatric meningitis has shown no survival advantage, but there is a reduction in the incidence of severe neurologic complications and deafness.

VIRAL MENINGITIS

Features of viral meningitis may be similar to bacterial meningitis. Cause could be all nonbacterial pathogens. Drugs, malignancies, and autoimmune diseases are other causes. Viral meningitis is treated by acyclovir given in dose of 10 mg/kg/IV. For patients with cytomegalovirus infection, ganciclovir is an alternative. Management of fungal and parasitic meningitis is detailed here.

BRAIN ABSCESS TREATMENT[4]

Brain abscess can arise from direct inoculation of infection following trauma, surgery, from spread of infection of ear or sinuses, or hematogenous spread from, e.g. lungs, heart (endocarditis). The condition may be nonspecific signs, neurological symptoms. The condition needs urgent investigation by computed tomography (CT)/magnetic resonance imaging (MRI) scan.

Causes include ear infections that may have mixed anaerobes, coliforms, etc. Sinuses may harbor pneumococci, streptococci that can lead to infections. Trauma/surgery may be associated with *Staphylococcus aureus* meningitis. Chest infections are related to *Staphylococcus* or pneumococci. Examination of pus aspirated from abscess is the main form of diagnostic tool. CSF, blood cultures can be done. Surgical drainage could be a priority. Antibiotics should be chosen with good penetration of CNS. Management consists of surgical treatment and antibiotics.

Cefotaxime 2 grams every 8 hourly is usually the first choice. Cotrimoxazole 5 mg/kg/IV given every 6 hourly can be another choice. Penicillin G-24 million units given IV divided into four doses can be given. Metronidazole can be given 1 g/IV followed by 500 mg every 5 hourly. Nafcillin 2 grams IV given every 4–6 hourly can be used for penetrating head trauma or neurosurgery. Chloramphenicol 100 mg/kg given 4–6 hourly could be given in patients with anaerobic infections. Chloramphenicol can be an alternative if allergy to beta-lactams.

TUBERCULAR MENINGITIS[5]

Tuberculous meningitis occurs most often in children and adults with immune compromise. The meningitis results from seeding of a tuberculoma in the brain or meninges. The tuberculoma, in turn, arises from the hematogenous spread from a primary focus in the lung. The patients present with headache, malaise, and fever. Weight loss may be prominent.

A physical examination may show normal results, or nuchal rigidity may be present. The CSF shows a moderate pleocytosis (usually fewer than 300 WBCs/ cubic mm), mostly lymphocytes. The level of protein is high and the amount of sugar low.

Acid-fast bacillus or AFB strains of the CSF can show presence of bacteria. Routine cultures are negative, but specialized cultures may take 4–8 weeks to grow. The chest X-ray and tuberculin skin test may be helpful, but both can show normal results. Polymerase chain reaction testing is rapid and fairly accurate. However, there can be false-negative findings if there are few organisms.

If the diagnosis of tuberculous meningitis is suspected on clinical grounds, treatment should be instituted. Isoniazid, streptomycin, rifampin, and pyrazinamide are used in combination. Ethambutol may be useful if given in high doses. Treatment is continued for at least 6–9 months. Corticosteroids may be helpful in reducing the inflammatory response, which itself can contribute to the patient's symptoms. Sequelae are common.

Tubercular meningitis has higher incidence in immigrant populations who come from countries with a higher incidence of TB (e.g. India, China) in the USA but in India, the problem is almost endemic. The disease has insidious onset and high frequency of complications, cranial nerve palsies. Delayed diagnosis makes complications more likely.

NEONATAL MENINGITIS

Group B streptococcus (*Streptococcus agalactiae*) and *Escherichia coli* are the principal causes. Bacteria travel via the bloodstream but direct infection may occur. Premature rupture of membranes, preterm delivery, or very low-birth weight babies are risk factors. High morbidity and mortality is the main complication. Clinical features can be nonspecific. Early onset Group B infection is more common than late onset disease. Other causes: *Listeria, Staphylococcus, Salmonella,* and other GNB. Treatment includes cephalosporin, or penicillin + aminoglycoside combination.

VIRAL MENINGITIS

This primarily affects children and young adults. Milder signs and symptoms may start as respiratory or intestinal infection then viremia. CSF shows raised lymphocyte count (50–200/cubic mm); protein and sugar usually normal. Full recovery expected.

Causes include enteroviruses, echovirus, Coxsackie A, B virus, polio, etc. Paramyxovirus includes mumps, Herpes simplex, varicella zoster virus (VZV), adenoviruses, arboviruses, lymphocytic choriomeningitis, human immunodeficiency virus (HIV), etc. Diagnosis is made by examination of CSF. Storage of blood samples at -70°C of CSF for subsequent virus isolation is needed. Additionally throat swab, stool, and paired sera can be used.

FUNGAL MENINGITIS

Cryptococcus neoformans is the main cause. HIV and immunosuppressed patients are at risk. The onset of headache, fever, and neck stiffness occurs insidiously. Diagnosis is made on CSF examination. It shows raised lymphocyte count, protein, low sugar, capsulate yeasts, and antigen can occur. Treatment with amphotericin B + flucytosine is recommended.

ENCEPHALITIS

Encephalitis affects children and adults mostly. The condition presents with a variety of symptoms and signs. Drowsiness, confusion, coma, fits, nerve palsies, and paresis are usual presenting symptoms. Encephalitis may have sequelae, e.g. memory loss, motor impairment, etc. Electroencephalography (EEG), brain scan, CSF examination, and brain biopsy may establish diagnosis. Causes include sporadic [Herpes simplex, mumps, VZV, Epstein-Barr virus (EBV), rabies] or epidemic (Togaviruses, e.g. Japanese B encephalitis, enteroviruses, etc.). Postinfectious could be caused by measles, rubella, and postvaccination. Measles is the most common type. Subacute sclerosing panencephalitis (SSPE) is a degenerative disease caused by measles.

Herpes Simplex Encephalitis

This is the most common cause of sporadic encephalitis in previously healthy individuals. There may be evidence of herpes infection of skin, mucosae. Causes include severe hemorrhagic encephalitis affecting temporal lobe, focal signs, and epilepsy features can occur. High mortality so treatment urgently needed with acyclovir. Other causes include VZV, mumps, rabies, mycoplasma pneumonia, rickettsiae, and *Toxoplasma,* etc.

Subacute Sclerosing Panencephalitis

This is a rare complication of measles infection. Usually it affects children. Intellectual impairment, involuntary movements are common features. High titers of measles antibody could be found. Brain biopsy shows measles virus. The treatment is symptomatic and the condition has fatal outcome.

PRION DISEASES

Prion diseases are neurodegenerative disorders and have long incubation periods. They present with slow progressive spongiform encephalopathy and have fatal outcome. Kuru originally occurred in New Guinea, due to cannibalism, eating human brain.

Sporadic Creutzfeldt-Jakob disease (CJD) is a rare degenerative disease in over 50s. Recipients of growth hormone are at increased risk, use of surgical instruments contaminated with prion protein. Prions are PrP proteins in abnormal configuration resistant to destruction. Mutations of genes encoding these proteins can be inherited.

Since no effective treatment is available, focus is on providing relief.

GUILLAIN-BARRÉ SYNDROME

This is a common infectious polyneuritis. Patients present with paraesthesiae, progressive weakness of limbs, and respiratory failure. High CSF protein is usual feature. The condition is postinfectious and various infections implicated include *Campylobacter*, EBV, *Mycoplasma*, etc. Recovery is likely to occur with supportive care.

Guillain-Barré Syndrome encompasses acute immune-mediated polyneuropathies and peripheral nerve myelin is target of an immune attack. The disease starts at level of nerve root conduction blocks and muscle weakness. Eventually the patients get widespread patchy demyelination increased paralysis. The disease starts as progressive, fairly symmetric muscle weakness. It typically starts in proximal legs and 10% develop weakness in face or arms. It is important to know that the severe respiratory muscle weakness may develop in up to 1/3 and oropharyngeal weakness in about half.

Absent or depressed deep tendon reflexes may be the presenting symptoms. Prominent severe pain in lower back could be another feature. It is common to have paresthesias in hands and feet. Dysautonomia is very common, tachycardia, urinary retention, hypertenison alternating with hypotension, paralytic ileus can occur.

Diagnosis is made using albuminocytologic dissociation or elevated CSF protein with normal WBC is seen in 80–90% patients. Electromyography (EMG) helps confirm diagnosis = prolonged or absent F waves.

One would have to monitor respiratory status closely as up to 1/3 patients may need ventilatory support. In severe cases, intrarterial monitoring may be needed due to blood pressure fluctuations. Neuropathic pain can be managed with gabapentin or carbamazepine. Intravenous immunoglobulin or IVIG is the mainstay of treatment and is typically given for 5 days at 0.4 g/kg/d. Plasmapheresis may need to be done (4–6 courses over 8–10 days). Glucocorticoids do not seem to have role in management.

CONGENITAL INFECTIONS

Intrauterine infections include *Toxoplasma*, rubella, cytomegalovirus, syphilis, etc. During birth infections like herpes simplex, hepatitis B and HIV can occur. Prevention is needed.

NEUROCYSTICERCOSIS[5]

Neurocysticercosis is the most common CNS parasitic infection and is usual cause of epilepsy in developing countries. Seizures are partial and brief but status epilepticus can occur in some cases. Headache, nausea, and vomiting can occur as well. Diagnosis is done by radiological techniques, e.g. CT or MRI and finding of scolex is considered diagnostic. Usual treatment is done using albendazole but cysts in ophthalmic and spinal area should not be medically treated. Albendazole is not effective in calcified lesions. Corticosteroids are used to reduce edema. Seizures respond to single antiepileptic drugs. Hydrocephalus, intracranial hypertension, and meningitis are common complications. Surgery is not commonly needed but management should be individualized.

The focus of initial medical therapy is control of seizures, edema, intracranial hypertension, or hydrocephalus, when one of these conditions is present. Under certain circumstances, a ventricular shunt or other neurosurgical procedure may be indicated if hydrocephalous is suspected. Anthelminthic therapy, kills viable cysts and provokes an inflammatory response, may actually increase symptoms acutely (admission may be needed or dexamethasone is given alongwith). Anthelminthic therapy is generally indicated for symptomatic patients with multiple, live (noncalcified) cysticerci. Anthelminthic treatment will not benefit patients with dead worms (calcified cysts). Concomitant administration of steroids (e.g. dexamethasone) is often indicated to suppress the inflammatory response induced by destruction of live cysticerci. Conventional anticonvulsant therapy is the mainstay of management of neurocysticercosis-associated seizure disorders. Albendazole in dose of 15 mg/kg/day in 2 divided doses for 15 days (prolonged course till 1 month or more may be needed) may be superior to praziquantel (50 mg/kg/day for 15 days) for the treatment of neurocysticercosis. Prolonged treatment courses (e.g. 30 days of albendazole, which may be repeated) may be needed.

NEUROSYPHILIS[5,6]

Syphilis can mimic infectious, vascular, neoplastic, or degenerative diseases. Meningitis may occur within

5 years of infection. After that, an inflammatory vasculitis (meningovascular syphilis) can produce infarction in virtually any area of the CNS. Tertiary syphilis (15–20 years after infection) has two classic presentations: (1) tabes dorsalis and (2) paretic neurosyphilis (general paresis of the insane).

Tabes dorsalis is an inflammatory process that affects the dorsal root ganglia, producing loss of position and vibration sensation, loss of deep-tendon reflexes, and severe "lightning" pains in the abdomen and legs. The Argyll Robertson pupil (light reaction lost but accommodation preserved) is usually present and bladder dysfunction is common.

General paresis consists of an infection of the cerebral cortex, particularly in the frontal lobes, producing a progressive frontal lobe dementia. Pupillary changes, myoclonic jerks, and tremor are also frequently present. Neurosyphilis may be diagnosed serologically using nonspecific (reagin) tests such as rapid plasma reagin (RPR) or Venereal Disease Research Laboratory (VDRL) test or specific treponemal antibody tests such as the fluorescent treponemal antibody (FTA) test. CSF pleocytosis or increased concentrations of CSF protein suggest active disease, treatment should be instituted. Prolonged treatment with penicillin is the treatment of choice.

CONCLUSION

Central nervous system infections usually have serious ramifications. Meningitis affects the membranes surrounding the brain and spinal cord and encephalitis affects the brain itself. Additionally, infections like neurocysticercosis can cause hydrocephalous seizures or motor manifestations. Likewise, fungal, viral and tubercular infections need urgent attention. Prompt diagnosis and treatment is mandatory.

REFERENCES

1. Riley Children's Health. (2017). Central nervous system infections. [online] Available from https://www.rileychildrens.org/health-info/central-nervous-system-infections. [Accessed May, 2018].
2. Parikh V, Tucci V, Galwankar S. Infections of the nervous system. Int J Crit Illn Inj Sci. 2012;2(2):82-97.
3. UpToDate. (2017). CNS infections. [online] Available from https://www.uptodate.com/contents/table-of-contents/infectious-diseases/cns-infections. [Accessed May, 2018].
4. Swenson R. (2017). Infectious diseases of the central nervous system. [online] Available from https://www.dartmouth.edu/~dons/part_3/chapter_25.html. [Accessed May, 2018].
5. Family Practice Notebook. (2017). CNS infections. [online] Available from https://www.fpnotebook.com/Neuro/ID/CnsInfctn.htm. [Accessed May, 2018].
6. Knudsen RP. (2017). Neurosyphilis: Overview of syphilis of the CNS. [online] Available from https://emedicine.medscape.com/article/1169231-overview. [Accessed May, 2018].

CHAPTER

16

Analgesics in Neurological Practice

DRUGS FOR MILD TO MODERATE PAIN: NONSTEROIDAL ANTI-INFLAMMATORY DRUGS

Millions of people worldwide use nonsteroidal anti-inflammatory drugs (NSAIDs) for pain, fever, and headache in neurology. NSAIDs like fenoprofen, ibuprofen, ketoprofen, naproxen, and naproxen sodium, are probably effective for migraine prevention.[1]

Lot of people with headache or backache uses these drugs on regular basis. NSAIDs are known as nonsteroidal as steroids too have powerful anti-inflammatory effect and this makes them different from steroids.

As on today, NSAIDs are among the most commonly used drugs worldwide for pain and fever. A complete understanding of their pharmacology is thus important to better prescribing or monitoring their side effects in patients. NSAIDs are usually regarded as drug with analgesic without impairing consciousness, antipyretic, and anti-inflammatory effects.

Mechanism of Pain Relief

Nonsteroidal anti-inflammatory drugs act by inhibiting inflammatory mechanisms in the body (e.g. prostaglandins). This can lead to reduction in swelling, e.g. joint pain and also fever.

Prostaglandins are produced by the cells, promote inflammation, pain and fever, blood clotting function of platelets, and protect the lining of the stomach from damaging effects of acid. There are two COX enzymes: COX-1 and COX-2. These enzymes help produce prostaglandins that promote inflammation, pain, and fever (Flowchart 16.1).

Pharmacokinetics

Nonsteroidal anti-inflammatory drugs are weak acids, pH 3–5, and well-absorbed from stomach and intestinal mucosa. They are protein bound in plasma (albumin) and are metabolized in the liver.

Uses of Nonsteroidal Anti-inflammatory Drugs

Nonsteroidal anti-inflammatory drugs vary in potency, duration, eliminated from body, and how strongly they inhibit COX-1 which is related to the tendency to cause ulcers and bleeding. The more an NSAID blocks COX-1, the greater to cause ulcers and promote bleeding; meaning COX-2 selective NSAIDs are safer in this regard (Box 16.1).

Individual Nonsteroidal Anti-inflammatory Drugs

Aspirin is the oldest NSAID and was obtained from bark of willow plant by Hoffman over a century back. The drug is still used extensively. It is used for the following:

- *Antiplatelet*: The drug is used in low dose and irreversibly blocks enzyme cyclooxygenase and

Flowchart 16.1: Mechanism of nonsteroidal anti-inflammatory drugs (NSAIDs). These drugs inhibit the key enzyme producing prostaglandins in the body. This could lead to reduction of inflammation, pain, and fever. Irreversible inhibition of this enzyme by aspirin can also lead to antiplatelet action. There are two kinds of cyclooxygenases enzymes producing prostaglandins in the body: (1) physiological (COX-1) and (2) pathological (COX-2). Former is responsible for constitutive roles, while latter is elevated in pathological situations.

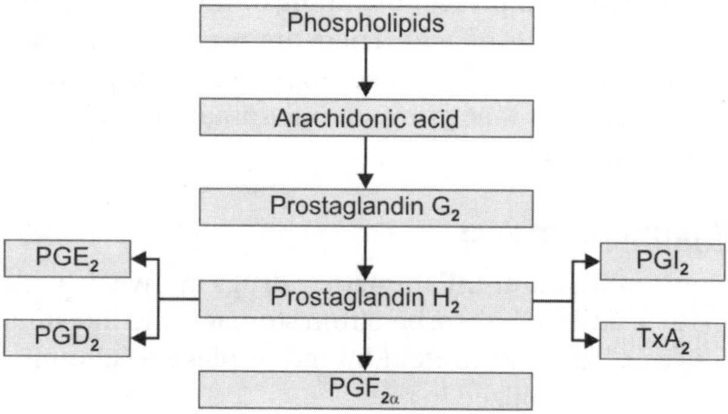

Box 16.1: Nonsteroidal anti-inflammatory drug (NSAID) uses.

- Rheumatoid arthritis
- Osteoarthritis
- Inflammatory arthritis
- Ankylosing spondylitis
- Psoriatic arthritis
- Reter's syndrome
- Acute gout
- Metastatic bone pain
- Dysmenorrhea
- Headache, migraine
- Postoperative pain
- Fever
- Paralytic ileus
- Renal colic.

achieves platelet inhibition. For this utility, it is prescribed extensively to those with myocardial infarction and stroke, etc.

- *Fever*: It is a routine antipyretic except in children.
- *Gout*: This is a common disorder of joints in which monosodium urate crystals accumulate. This leads to pain in great toes. Aspirin lowers uric acid and can treat an attack of acute gout.
- *Pain*: It has long been a useful agent in rheumatoid arthritis and juvenile rheumatoid arthritis. However, NSAIDs are useful in mild to moderate pain of bodily origin. In severe pain, opioids are used.

Topical Nonsteroidal Anti-inflammatory Drugs

Nonsteroidal anti-inflammatory drugs have good deal of topical activity, e.g. diclofenac, ibuprofen, and piroxicam. The drugs could be used in cervical spondylosis, low back pain, sprains, contusions, etc. Several topical preparations, e.g. gels, patches, and sprays are available for rapid relief nowadays.

Contraindications of Aspirin

It should not be used in:

- *Children with viral fever*: These are prone to develop a rare syndrome of hepatic encephalopathy called Rye's syndrome. As a general rule, aspirin is not used in children with viral fever below 11 years of age.
- *Peptic ulcer*: Since aspirin and other drugs have acidic nature, therefore, they remain soluble in acidic pH of stomach. Therefore, these could get concentrated in stomach cells. Moreover, these could also block production of protective prostaglandins leading to formation of ulcer known as peptic ulcer (Fig. 16.1).

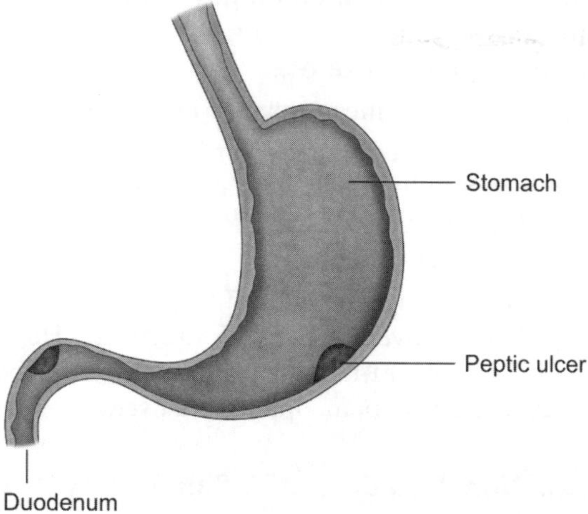

Fig. 16.1: Peptic ulcer involves punched out hole in cell membrane of mucosa of stomach. Therefore, there could be pain and loss of appetite. Nonsteroidal anti-inflammatory drugs (NSAIDs) are common causes of peptic ulcers.

- *Bleeding diathesis*: Patients with bleeding diseases are prone to development of hemorrhages due to antiplatelet nature of these drugs especially aspirin.
- *Asthma and related diseases*: Bronchial asthma and patients with Hey fever or those with nasobronchial allergy or nasal polyp are prone to development of bronchospasm. Therefore, NSAIDs should not be used in asthmatic patients.

Para-aminophenols

- Paracetamol (also called acetaminophen).
- Wherever aspirin is not used, paracetamol can be used. This is a para-aminophenol and is most widely used analgesic and antipyretic. It is especially useful to relieve pain of osteoarthritis. In neurology,

paracetamol is commonly used in tension headache and migraine.

- Propionic acid derivatives.

Ibuprofen

This is a safer older NSAID and is used for backache, posttraumatic pain, and menstrual-related pain. Some evidence suggests that it can reduce risk of dementia and Parkinson's disease. The drug has been shown to suppress plaque pathology in Alzheimer's disease dementia.

Flurbiprofen

This is used as a meiosis preventing agent during cataract. It is also used for rheumatoid arthritis, osteoarthritis, and other mild to moderate pain. Like ibuprofen, the drug has been shown to suppress plaque pathology and lower Abeta42 in Alzheimer's disease dementia mouse model.

Ketoprofen

This is one more propionic acid derivative and is used in arthritis-related pains. It should not be used for long term as use more than 5 days is associated with nephrotoxicity. Ketoprofen is used in acute migraine.

Arylacetic Acid

Diclofenac is commonly used drug of this class. It is not just used orally but also intramuscularly and topically. Studies have shown that when it is applied topically, then also there is sufficient blood levels reached. Moreover, risk of side effect via topical application as cream or ointment is less. It is used in sprains, muscle spasms, backache, and also in joint pains such as osteoarthritis or rheumatoid arthritis. Intramuscular injection is given post-traumatically and postoperatively.

Aceclofenac is a newer drug and is supposed to be equally or more effective compared to diclofenac. The drug has a high degree of selectivity for cyclooxygenase enzyme and is almost a COX-2 inhibitor.

Aceclofenac has significant analgesic and anti-inflammatory effect with good tolerance. The drug has low occurrence of gastrointestinal adverse reactions and higher adherence to treatment of chronic diseases. The drug is used extensively in acute and chronic low backache with or without thiocolchicoside, skeletal muscle relaxant.

Indoleacetic Acid

Indomethacin is most commonly used drug of this class. This is a potent and long-acting drug. It undergoes elimination by bile and is reabsorbed (enterohepatic circulation). This makes it longer acting.
It is the drug of choice for:

- *Acute attack of gout*: A joint disorder involving great toes.
- *Closure of ductus arteriosus*: Sometimes, after birth, there are intact communications between pulmonary artery and aorta which needs to be closed surgically. The drug, by inhibiting prostaglandin synthesis can close it.
- *Sexuality-associated headache*: Headaches can be associated with sexual activity and can be treated by indomethacin before sexual intercourse. It has also been used in paroxysmal hemicranias.
- *Ankylosing spondylitis*: This is a disorder of young males with genetic basis. Patients present with low backache and have bamboo spine. In later cases, even whole of spine gets involved and there can be breathing difficulty.

Side effects include frontal headache in about half of treated patients. Drug can also cause confusion, hence is avoided in:

- Psychiatric patients
- Epileptics
- Highway truck drivers.

Oxicams

Piroxicam and meloxicam were once popular; nowadays not so much. Better NSAIDs have become available now hence are used less commonly. Both of them are now available as topical ointments. It has been used topically in acute and chronic cervical and lower back pain.

Fenamates

Drugs like mefenamic acid are used extensively in gynecological and obstetrical cases to relieve uterine spasm associated with menstruation. Combinations of mefenamic acid with dicyclomine are available.

Fenamates are N-phenylanthranilic acid derivatives. The drugs have high efficacy but due to high incidence of adverse reactions they are used only for the treatment of acute painful states. Tolfenamic acid, meclofenamic acid, flufenamic acid, and etofenamic acid are other examples.

Pyrrolopyrrole

Ketorolac is a very potent NSAID and is used for moderately severe acute pain that usually requires narcotics. Ketorolac causes ulcers more frequently than other NSAID. Therefore, it is not used for more than 5 days. Individuals who do not respond to one NSAID may respond to another. Ketorolac has been tried in tension type headache and has been most commonly used parenteral NSAID in USA for acute treatment of neurological emergencies involving pain, e.g. migraine.

Cyclooxygenase-2 Inhibitors

As stated earlier, COX-2 enzyme is pathological and plays a vital role in cell adhesion, migration, and oxidative burst, i.e. in steps needed for cellular inflammation.

Celecoxib was the first of this group of drugs and is still used widely in joint disorders such as rheumatoid or osteoarthritis. Data indicates that celecoxib can improve cognitive profile.

Rofecoxib and valdecoxib were banned in 2002 and 2004, respectively. Former was banned due to adverse cardiovascular events, while latter due to high incidence of allergic reactions.

Nonsteroidal Anti-inflammatory Drugs Poisonings

Young children are particularly affected and may consume large number of aspirin or paracetamol tablets.

- *Aspirin poisoning*: Aspirin in large dose can interfere with respiration and can cause respiratory acidosis in children. In adults, metabolic acidosis occurs later. Treatment involves using vitamin K and fresh frozen plasma. Hemodialysis can be used in severe cases.
- *Paracetamol poisoning*: Children with paracetamol ingestion (especially after ingesting 10–15 tablets) can come with liver enlargement and jaundice. Hepatocellular failure and death may occur. Within 24 hours, an antidote acetylcysteine is given. If this fails, then even liver transplant may be needed.

Long-term Side Effects of Nonsteroidal Anti-inflammatory Drugs Therapy

- *Cardiovascular*: A significant increase in acute myocardial infarction (AMI) risk with newer COX-2 can occur and this is more than high dose of traditional NSAID. Likewise, there is a heart failure risk also.

- *Gastrointestinal*: Direct irritation due to acidic molecules is a common problem. Indirect irritation due to inhibition of COX-1 reduces protective prostaglandins. This can manifest as nausea, vomiting, dyspepsia, gastric ulcer/bleeding, diarrhea, etc. depending upon duration of therapy and dose.
- *Renal*: Decrease prostaglandins → constriction of afferent arteriole → decreased renal perfusion → alters renal function. This presents as salt and fluid retention, hypertension. NSAID with angiotensin converting enzyme (ACE) inhibitor, diuretic should be monitored. Rare side effects such as acute renal failure (ARF), acute tubular necrosis (ATN), and nephrotic syndromes can also occur.
- *Allergic*: Allergy, shortness of breath, or precipitation or worsening of asthma—a higher risk for serious allergic reaction can occur. Patients with a serious allergy to one NSAID are likely to have similar reaction to a different NSAID.
- *Combinational risks*: Allergy, shortness of breath, or precipitation or worsening of asthma—a higher risk for serious allergic reaction can occur. Patients with a serious allergy to one NSAID are likely to have similar reaction to a different NSAID.
- *Pregnancy*: Nonsteroidal anti-inflammatory drugs are not recommended during pregnancy, particular 3rd trimester. NSAIDs can cause early closure of fetal ductus arteriosus and fetal renal toxicity, premature birth. Acetaminophen is more safe during pregnancy.

Choosing Nonsteroidal Anti-inflammatory Drugs

All NSAIDs have similar mechanism of action—inhibition of eicosanoids synthesis (with higher or lower selectivity and strength). NSAIDs differ in the strength of COX1/COX2 inhibition and the incidence of typical adverse effects, e.g. ulcer disease, bleeding, etc. The usual dose of aspirin, for example are given here:

- *Antipyretic*: 600 mg
- *Analgesic*: 600 mg (4–6 hours)
- *Antirheumatic, uricosuric*: 3–6 g/day
- *Antiplatelet*: 30–300 mg.

Management of Nonsteroidal Anti-inflammatory Drugs-induced Side Effects

Dose reduction can be helpful or the drugs can be changed. Combination of NSAIDs with protective drugs, e.g. proton pump inhibitors such as lansoprazole, or omeprazole can be used. Prostaglandin analogs such as misoprostol or H_2 antihistamines—cimetidine, ranitidine, and famotidine can be used. Antacids can be quick solution as well. One can chose selective COX-2 inhibitors as well.

OPIOIDS[2]

Sir William Osler, father of medicine was once so impressed with morphine, that he called it the "God's own medicine".

Morphine is a plant-derived drug and is used for a variety of situations. It is obtained from juice of poppy plant (Fig. 16.2). It was isolated over 200 years back and is still isolated from plants.

Mechanism

The drug acts by reducing the release of pain producing substance in the brain and spinal cord and this raised pain threshold (Fig. 16.3). This is considered to be their major pharmacological action.

Pharmacokinetics

Opioids are lipid soluble hence, have excellent oral absorption. These are extensively metabolized in liver.

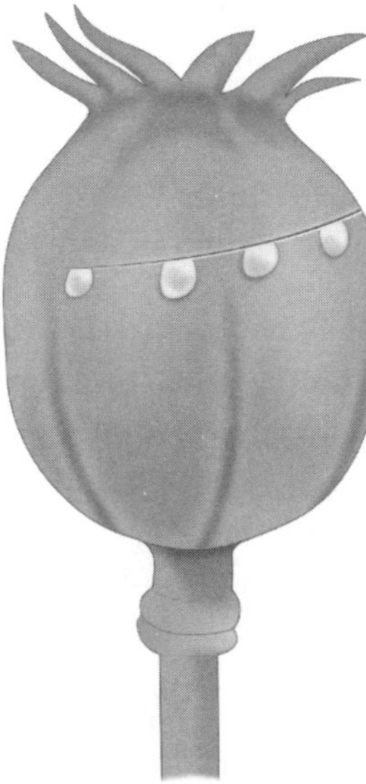

Fig. 16.2: Morphine is obtained from juice of poppy plant. The juice is dried and drugs like morphine, codeine, thebaine, and papaverine are obtained.

Remifentanil is shortest acting and buprenorphine is longest-acting opioid.

Some opioids like sufentanil and alfentanil are protein bound. Codeine is a prodrug and forms morphine in the body. Similarly, pethidine forms norpethidine that can accumulate in renal failure patient leading to even development of seizure activity.

Pharmacological Actions

Brain

Opioids reduce anxiety and produce sedation. Analgesia and euphoria occurs, high dose can cause respiratory depression. Nausea and vomiting occurs due to

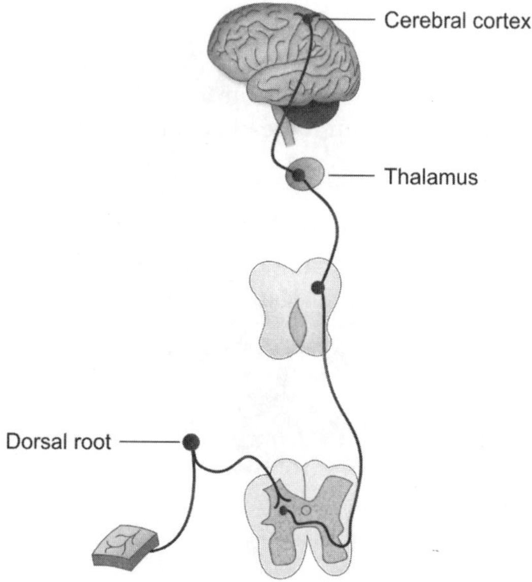

Fig. 16.3: Drugs of opioid class stimulate G-protein coupled receptors and cause cellular hyperpolarization. There are three types of opioid receptors: (1) mu, (2) kappa, and (3) delta. All mediate analgesia. Analgesia by these receptors is exhibited both at the level of brain and spinal cord.

stimulation of central centers. Prolonged use can lead to abuse and dependence. Cough is suppressed and intracranial tension becomes high.

Prolonged use can produce endocrinal alterations leading to reduced release of growth hormone and increase in release of prolactin. This can cause impotence or interference with reproductive functions.

Reduced body temperature can occur in overdose.

Face

Facial and lip swelling can occur.

Bronchi

Bronchi become constricted and this can be very harmful in patients with asthma. In acute asthma, if morphine is given, it can lead even to death. So, the drug must not be given.

Chest

Mu receptor-mediated chest wall rigidity can occur and this can interfere with ventilator functions. "Armor chest" is a manifestation.

Lungs

Differential vasodilatation occurs. Blood vessels of body are dilated and therefore, blood shifts from lungs to systemic circulation. This makes them very useful for treatment of acute pulmonary edema.

Gut

There is an increase in activity of circular muscles and reduction in activity of longitudinal muscles. Tolerance to this constipating action does not occur and even habitual addicts remain constipated. There can be contraction of sphincter of Oddi. This can precipitate an attack of biliary colic.

Urinary Tract

There is contraction of ureter, and also that of urinary bladder. Urinary retention occurs as along with detrusor contraction; bladder neck also contracts.

Uses

Morphine is used for:
- Pulmonary edema
- Cancer pain

- Pain of terminal illness
- Tetralogy of Fallot.

Routine use of opioids in neurological indications, e.g. headache, low back pain, etc. is not recommended as the benefit outweighs the risk.[3,4]

Pethidine

Pethidine and pentazocine is used in visceral pain. The drug does not have any particular utility in neurological disorders but is sometimes used to treat cancer pain. It can interfere with papillary assessment if it has been given in head injury.

Methadone

It is used for opioid addicts and is used for those who become dependent upon these drugs and cannot live without. Buprenorphine is a longer-acting drug that can also be used for same reason. Methadone is used as an analgesic also.

Codeine

This is often used in cough and cold mixtures. It also is very useful to treat cancer pain and diarrheas. Codeine has significant abuse potential with withdrawal. Dextromethorphan is a synthetic drug and is used as a cough suppressant. It does not cause constipation like codeine and has significantly less abuse potential.

Naltrexone

This is most potent opioid antagonist and is used to reduce alcohol craving and also for treating impotence. It has been found to have anti-inflammatory effects as well. Naltrexone has been tried in multiple sclerosis as well.

Naloxone

This is a commonly used opioid antagonist and is given intravenously for opioid overdose. It is a short-acting drug, hence redistribution occurs quickly. It is also used in hepatic coma. If a mother during pregnancy has been given high dose of opioids, then naloxone can be given to newborn baby in his/her umbilical vein and this can reverse neonatal depression.

Contraindications

- *Head injury*: Do not use opioids in head injury as they cause respiratory depression and this can cause increase in intracranial tension.
- *Asthma*: Bronchospasm occurs.
- *Hypotension*: Do not use opioids as it gets aggravated.
- *Biliary colic*: Since opioids can cause spasm of sphincter of Oddi, these are not used in biliary colic. Since, pethidine is less likely to provoke spasm this can still be used.
- *Benign enlargement of prostate*: In these patients, opioids increase the problem as these can cause urinary retention.

CONCLUSION

Nonsteroidal anti-inflammatory drugs (NSAIDs) have been in use for many years in general medicine and constitute a large part of prescriptions issued in daily practice. Although NSAIDs are used for many diseases in neurology, they have also been tested as a new therapeutic option for various other diseases. While their effects on headache and cerebrovascular diseases are well known, little is known about their impact on neurodegenerative diseases. A trial of indomethacin had shown some protective effect in Alzheimer's disease. NSAIDs have long been the mainstay of treatment of migraine and many other forms of headaches. Aspirin is used commonly in stroke prophylaxis. The long-term use of NSAIDs is fraught with several side effects and need to be monitored for better safety.[5,6]

REFERENCES

1. Holland S, Silberstein SD, Freitag F, et al. Evidence-based guideline update: NSAIDs and other complementary treatments for episodic migraine prevention in adults: report of the Quality Standards Subcommittee of the American Academy of Neurology and the American Headache Society. Neurology. 2012;78(17):1346-53.
2. Franklin GM, American Academy of Neurology. Opioids for chronic noncancer pain: a position paper of the American Academy of Neurology. Neurology. 2014;83(14):1277-84.
3. American Academy of Neurology (AAN) (2017). Opioid therapies. [online] Available from https://www.aan.com/policy-and-guidelines/quality/public-health/opioid-therapies/. [Accessed May, 2018].
4. Markman J, Narasimhan SK (2017). Treatment of pain. [online] Available from https://www.msdmanuals.com/professional/neurologic-disorders/pain/treatment-of-pain. [Accessed May, 2018].
5. Terzi M, Altun G, Şen S, et al. The use of non-steroidal anti-inflammatory drugs in neurological diseases. J Chem Neuroanat. 2018 Jan;87:12-24. doi: 10.1016/j.jchemneu.2017.03.003. Epub 2017 Mar 21.
6. Holland S1, Silberstein SD, Freitag F, et al. Quality Standards Subcommittee of the American Academy of Neurology and the American Headache Society. Evidence-based guideline update: NSAIDs and other complementary treatments for episodic migraine prevention in adults: report of the Quality Standards Subcommittee of the American Academy of Neurology and the American Headache Society.Neurology. 2012 Apr 24;78(17):1346-53. doi: 10.1212/WNL.0b013e3182535d0c.

CHAPTER

17

Drug Treatment of Complex Regional Pain Syndrome

HISTORY

During World War, it was seen that a chronic pain syndrome in soldiers who suffered traumatic nerve injuries. Their symptoms included constant burning pain and significant trophic changes. This syndrome was described as *causalgia* (from the Greek *kausis—burning* and *algos—pain*).

Half a century later, a French surgeon named René Leriche implicated the sympathetic nervous system in causalgic pain. He treated these patients with surgical sympathectomy.[1] In the 1950s, John Bonica introduced the phrase *reflex sympathetic dystrophy* (RSD) after noticing the efficacy of temporary blockade of the sympathetic nervous system in these patients.

TERMINOLOGY

There have since been many confusing terms used to describe the condition (Box 17.1).[2]

Box 17.1: Terminologies used to define complex regional pain syndrome.[2]

- Acute atrophy of the bone
- Algodystrophy
- Algoneurodystrophy
- Chronic traumatic edema
- Postinfarctional sclerodactyly
- Post-traumatic algodystrophy
- Post-traumatic dystrophy
- Post-traumatic osteoporosis
- Post-traumatic spreading neuralgia
- Post-traumatic sympathetic dystrophy
- Pseudodystrophy
- Reflex neurovascular dystrophy
- Shoulder hand syndrome
- Sudeck's dystrophy
- Sympathalgia
- Traumatic angiospasm
- Traumatic vasospasm.

INTERNATIONAL SOCIETY OF STUDY OF PAIN DEFINITION[3]

In 1993, the International Association for the Study of Pain (IASP) introduced the term *complex regional pain syndrome* (CRPS) to describe all pain states that previously would have been diagnosed as RSD or causalgia-like syndromes.

As per IASP, CRPS is:

- *Complex*: Varied and dynamic clinical presentation.
- *Regional*: Nondermatomal distribution of symptoms.
- *Pain*: Out of proportion to the inciting events.
- *Syndrome*: Constellation of symptoms and signs.
- The term "sympathetic" was avoided in the revised definition because its contribution is not constant across patients.

- Complex regional pain syndrome pain may be "sympathetically maintained pain" (SMP) or "sympathetically independent pain" (SIP).
- Complex regional pain syndrome can be separated into two types based on the presence or absence of a nerve injury:
    1. *Complex regional pain syndrome type I*: A syndrome that develops after an initiating noxious event that may or may not be associated with a period of immobilization.
    2. *Complex regional pain syndrome type II*: Differs from CRPS type I by the presence of a known injury to a nerve or nerves.

CLINICAL FEATURES[4,5]

Characteristic triad of symptoms comprising *autonomic*, *sensory*, and *motor* disturbances. Triad given earlier, however, can differ amongst individuals. Symptoms will generally change over time in a given individual. Distal edema and skin temperature changes are found in majority of patients. The affected area is initially warm, but over the course of the disease the skin temperature decreases. Skin becomes red initially and becomes pale in the chronic disease. Altered sweating can occur and increased sweating more common. Nail and hair changes can occur and there can be increased growth in early disease.

Other features include: spontaneous pain, often described as burning, aching, throbbing, shooting, or deep pressure pain. Hyperpathia and hyperalgesia are common and allodynia can occur as well. Motor changes, e.g. weakness, distal tremors, dystonia, and myoclonus occur as well.

It is not clear whether these are part of the clinical presentation of the disease or a result of protection/

disuse of the painful limb. Osteoporosis and joint stiff can occur late in the course of disease.

Patients often have associated psychological and psychiatric disturbances. These are generally consequences of the disorder rather than causes thereof.

PATHOPHYSIOLOGY[5,6]

Three main hypotheses have been proposed to explain the abnormalities in CRPSs:

1. Facilitated neurogenic inflammation.
2. Autonomic dysfunction.
3. Neuroplastic changes within the central nervous system (CNS).

Neurogenic Inflammation

This hypothesis is substantiated by the fact that the classic inflammatory signs are present in CRPS, e.g. pain, swelling, erythema, hyperthermia, and impaired function. However, when clinical chemistry parameters for inflammation are evaluated, there are no differences between CRPS patients and controls. With neurogenic inflammation, distinct classes of C-fibers called mechano-heat insensitive C-fibers have both an afferent function in the mediation of pain and itch as well as an efferent neurosecretory function, releasing neuropeptides via "axon reflex". Action potentials in these fibers can be conducted retrogradely to terminal branches via axon collaterals where neuropeptides such as substance P and calcitonin gene-related peptide (CGRP) are released. Substance P provokes plasma protein extravasation (edema) and appears to have a role in osteoclastic activity. CGRP induces vasodilation (hyperthermia and erythema), increases sweating, and appears to be involved in hair growth.

Autonomic Dysfunction

Pathological Sympatho-afferent Coupling

Peripheral nociceptors develop adrenergic sensitivity (mainly alpha-2 receptors) such that tonic sympathetic efferent activity leads to their activation. Painful impulses via these nociceptors maintain the CNS in a sensitized state. Painful and nonpainful stimuli to the affected limb result in hyperalgesia and allodynia, respectively. Catecholamine levels, however, are actually lower in the affected extremity, thus, it is not a problem of excessive sympathetic nerve output.

Neuroplastic Changes within the Central Nervous System

Studies using functional brain imaging in patients with CRPS have found a significant degree of cortical reorganization in the central sensory and motor cortices. The amount of reorganization positively correlates with the extent of pain intensity. The areas of reorganization were found to be reversible in adequately treated patients.

DIAGNOSIS

The diagnosis is based exclusively on the characteristic clinical features of the condition.

International Association for the Study of Pain Diagnostic Criteria for Complex Regional Pain Syndrome

- Presence of an initiating noxious event or cause of immobilization.
- Continuing pain, allodynia, or hyperalgesia, with pain disproportionate to any inciting event.

- Evidence at sometime of edema, changes in skin blood flow, or abnormal sudomotor activity in the region of pain.
- Diagnosis is excluded by the existence of conditions that would otherwise account for the degree of pain and dysfunction.

Differential Diagnosis

- Unrecognized local pathology (fracture, sprain)
- Traumatic vasospasm
- Cellulitis
- Lymphedema
- Raynaud's disease
- Thromboangiitis obliterans
- Erythromelalgia
- Deep vein thrombosis (DVT)
- Also, nerve entrapment syndromes, occupational overuse syndromes, and diabetic neuropathy.

Apart from clinical history, general physical and detailed neurological examination, plain radiographs, X-ray bone densitometry, and magnetic resonance imaging have not been shown to be sensitive or specific for CRPS. Bone uptake studies could be done.

TREATMENT

The primary aim of treating patients is to reduce pain, swelling, and improve quality of life. Several drug class/s or combinations are useful for treatment. Many interventional methods and nonpharmacological approaches are used alone or in combination with each other for successful management.

- *Sympathetic ganglia blockade*:
  - *Stellate ganglion*: Upper extremities
  - *Lumbar paravertebral ganglia*: Lower extremities.

Evaluation of the effects of the block on sudomotor and vasoconstrictor function by assessing skin blood flow, temperature, and resistance is vitally important to know whether the sympathetic block is complete, especially in patients who do not experience significant pain relief.

Local anesthetic can spread to nearby nerve roots, resulting in somatic nerve block that may significantly affect the patient's pain. Therefore, it is important to do a careful sensory examination of the affected area. If a large dose of local anesthetics is used, systemic uptake may provide some pain relief.

The invasive procedure itself may have a significant placebo effect. Visceral sensory afferent fibers traveling with the sympathetic chain may be blocked and result in pain relief.

- *Regional intravenous block with guanethidine*: Guanethidine is an antihypertensive drug class. Drug taken up by postganglionic sympathetic nerves where it depletes norepinephrine stores and prevents further release of norepinephrine for 1–2 days. The initial depletion of norepinephrine stores can cause short-term excitation of nociceptors due to the increased norepinephrine release leading to increased pain during the procedure.
  - *Pharmacotherapy*: A multidisciplinary approach utilizing pharmacotherapy, physical therapy, and psychological therapy is most appropriate. Several drugs have been demonstrated to be effective for CRPS based on randomized controlled trials.

    Tricyclic antidepressants, e.g. amitriptyline are used widely in patients with neuropathic pain. They are currently the best drugs to treat neuropathic pain.[7] Antidepressants of this class work by a variety of mechanisms, and in the end reduce posterior horn hyperactivity.

Prednisone given orally is an anti-inflammatory and neuronal membrane stabilizer. They are beneficial for patients who present with redness, swelling, and heat.[8]

Vitamin C is used as an antioxidant. Alendronate is given intravenously (IV) and is an osteoclast inhibitor.

Bretylium is given IV as an autonomic ganglia blocker. Ketanserin given IV has been tried as a serotonin and alpha receptor antagonist. Likewise, phentolamine given IV acts as an alpha-1 receptor antagonist. Lidocaine blocks sodium channels and is a very popular local anesthetic. Calcitonin given intranasally is tried as an osteoclast inhibitor.

Clonidine[9] given epidurally has been used as an alpha-2 receptor agonist to reduce sympathetic activity (sympatholytic activity). Baclofen[10] as oral or intrathecal is used as a gamma-aminobutyric acid-B (GABA-B) receptor agonist to reduce spasticity.

Antiepileptics, antidepressants, ketamine, nonsteroidal anti-inflammatory drugs (NSAIDs), and/or opioids have been tried from time to time.[11]

- *Physiotherapy*:[12] Early physical therapy is essential to avoid atrophy and contractures of the affected limb. Physiotherapy with or without occupational therapy have been shown to reduce pain and motor impairment, and improve function and coordination ability of the limb. Importantly, this requires that the patient take an active role in their care.
- *Psychosocial interventions*: Such interventions are an integral part of the multidisciplinary treatment approach. Many patients with CRPSs have a significant amount of psychological dysfunction, which is a reflection of the disease process itself

as opposed to a cause thereof. Pain coping skills, biofeedback, relaxation training, cognitive behavioral therapy, and mirror therapy have been tried.

- *Interventional*: Sympathetic nerve blocks are used both as diagnostic and therapeutic tools. These are also useful for helping patients tolerate physical and occupational therapy. Effectiveness of repeat blocks may, however, be unpredictable. If a plateau of responsiveness to these blocks is reached, more advanced interventional therapies may need to be considered.
- *Cord stimulation*:[13] Spinal cord stimulation has been shown to be effective in randomized controlled trials that have demonstrated a significant reduction in level of pain and improvement in functional status and quality-of-life in patients with cord stimulation plus physical therapy compared to those undergoing physical therapy alone.
- *Surgical/chemical sympathectomy*: Surgical sympathectomy appears significantly more effective than chemical sympathectomy. There is, however, considerable risk of developing a postsympathectomy pain syndrome that may be the result of a denervation supersensitivity of alpha receptors. Peripheral nerve stimulation has been tried as well.

RECENT ADVANCES

- *Intravenous immunoglobulin (IVIG)* has been shown to be effective in small trials of patients who had not responded to other treatment. Significantly, more decrease in pain scores occurred in these patients.
- *Ketamine*: In unresponsive pain, low dose ketamine has been tried.
- *Graded motor imagery*: This is a new technique that has been tried in patients unresponsive to everything.

CONCLUSION

Complex regional pain syndrome is a complicated chronic pain syndrome with variable clinical presentation and complicated diagnostic criteria. Diagnosis is made on a clinical basis and treatment is best managed with a multidisciplinary approach including medications, interventional procedures, physical therapy, and psychological therapy.

REFERENCES

1. National Institute of Neurological Disorders and Stroke (NINDS). (2017). Chronic regional pain syndrome: Factsheet. [online] Available from https://www.ninds.nih.gov/Disorders/Patient-Caregiver-Education/Fact-Sheets/Complex-Regional-Pain-Syndrome-Fact-Sheet. [Accessed May, 2018].
2. Wheeler AH. (2018). An overview of complex regional pain syndromes. [online] Available from https://emedicine.medscape.com/article/1145318-overview. [Accessed May, 2018].
3. National Health Trust Choices. (2017). Complex regional pain syndrome: an overview. [online] Available from https://www.nhs.uk/conditions/complex-regional-pain-syndrome/. [Accessed May, 2018].
4. Pain Australia. (2017). Complex regional pain syndrome. [online] Available from https://www.painaustralia.org.au/about-pain/forms-of-pain/complex-regional-pain-syndrome. [Accessed May, 2018].
5. FamilyDoctor.org. (2017). Complex regional pain syndrome. [online] Available from https://familydoctor.org/condition/complex-regional-pain-syndrome/. [Accessed May, 2018].
6. Markman J, Narasimhan SK. (2017). Complex regional pain syndrome. [online] Available from https://www.merckmanuals.com/professional/neurologic-disorders/pain/complex-regional-pain-syndrome-crps. [Accessed May, 2018].

7. Netherlands Society of Rehabilitation Specialists. (2014). Updated guidelines for complex regional pain syndrome type 1. [online] Available from http://pdver.atcomputing.nl/pdf/Executive_summary_guideline_CRPS_I_2014_docx.pdf. [Accessed May, 2018].
8. Barbalinardo S, Loer SA, Goebel A, et al. The treatment of long-standing complex regional pain syndrome with oral steroids. Pain Med. 2016;17(2):337-43.
9. Mackey S, Feinberg S. Pharmacologic therapies for complex regional pain syndrome. Curr Pain Headache Rep. 2007;11(1):38-43.
10. Wheeler AH. (2018). Complex regional pain syndromes: Treatment and management. [online] Available from https://emedicine.medscape.com/article/1145318-treatment. [Accessed May, 2018].
11. Chung OY, Bruehl S. (2003). Complex regional pain syndrome. [online] Available from http://rsds.org/wp-content/uploads/2015/02/chung.pdf. [Accessed May, 2018].
12. Pollard C. (2013). Physiotherapy management of complex regional pain syndrome. [online] Available from https://rsds.org/wp-content/uploads/2015/05/ICC-Pollard.pdf. [Accessed May, 2018].
13. Shrivastav M, Musley S. Spinal cord stimulation for complex regional pain syndrome. Conf Proc IEEE Eng Med Biol Soc. 2009;2009:2033-6.

CHAPTER

18

Treatment of Cerebral Palsy

INTRODUCTION

As per Indian Academy of Pediatrics (Neurology chapter), cerebral palsy is a nonspecific term that include disorders characterized by early onset and impaired movement and posture. This is a nonprogressive condition and may include perceptual problems, language deficits, and intellectual involvement.[1]

Cerebral palsy is chronic disability of central nervous system origin characterized by aberrant control of movement of posture, appearing early in life, and not the result of progressive neurological disease.[2]

INCIDENCE

Number wise, this is the most common physical disability of childhood. Incidence has increased since in the last 50 years, may be due to improved survival of very low-birth weight babies.[1]

ETIOLOGY[1]

A variety of perinatal, prenatal, and postnatal factors contribute, either singly or multifactorily to cerebral palsy. Traditionally, it is thought to be due to birth asphyxia; now known to be due to existing prenatal brain abnormalities. Premature delivery is the single most important determinant of cerebral palsy. In a significant percentage, however, no cause may be found as well.[1]

Cerebral palsy is a group of neuromuscular disorders resulting from damage primarily to the motor region of the brain, causing impairment in control over voluntary muscles. It is not hereditary and may occur through anoxia (lack of oxygen during birth). It is one of the commonest neurodevelopmental disorders seen in neurological/pediatric clinics.

CLINICAL FEATURES[2-4]

The majority of children with cerebral palsy are born with it, although it may not be detected until months or years later. The early signs of cerebral palsy usually appear before a child reaches 3 years of age.

Symptoms include a birth history of prematurity, seizures, and/or intracranial hemorrhage. Delayed milestones are common. Periventricular leukomalacia could be found on magnetic resonance imaging (MRI) brain.

Abnormal motor performance is usual on neurological examination. Muscle tone may be altered and child could be spastic with persistence of primitive reflexes. Posture may be abnormal. Mental retardation could be present with speech delay or dysarthria. Vision and hearing may be affected. Behavior abnormalities are common with or without learning difficulties.

Very young patients can present with feeding problems, failure to suck breast milk, tongue trusting, gagging, and choking. Vomiting and regurgitation with dribbling and constipation is common.

Crying, screaming, and sleep disturbances often result. Most may have growth retardation as well.

Types of cerebral plasies are outlined in Table 18.1.

MANAGEMENT[2-6]

- *General*: Parent guidance and education is a must.
- *Physiotherapy*: Regular physiotherapy is helpful. This is the most commonly used treatment. The treatment goal is to develop good skeletal alignment for the spastic child. For the child with athetosis, training in purposeful acts, even in the face of involuntary motion could be an acceptable aim. Maximum development of proprioceptive sense for the child with ataxia should be there. Orthotic devices (braces, splints, casting, etc.) could be used.
- *Orthopedic*: Orthopedic abnormalities may need corrections. Orthopedic surgery may be needed to correct contractures or spastic deformities. This may be important to provide stability for uncontrolled joint. Also, this may be able to provide balanced muscle power.
- *Speech and occupational therapy:* From time to time, they may be needed as well. Training in activates of daily living along with developmental lines could be

TABLE 18.1: Types of cerebral palsies.

- Spastic cerebral palsy—causes stiffness and movement difficulties.
- *Dyskinetic:* which can be either *athetoid cerebral palsy*—leads to involuntary and uncontrolled movements or *ataxic cerebral palsy*—causes a disturbed sense of balance and depth perception.
- *Mixed:* this is a mixture of different types of cerebral palsy. A common combination is spastic and athetoid.

useful. Sitting to walking, feeding to cooking could be taught. It is important to incorporate play into program so that it is not perceived as hectic. Adaptive equipment, e.g. utensils for functional use, i.e. eating, writing should be taught.

Early speech training by speech/language pathologist is needed. Before child develops poor habits, such training should be started. One should always advice parents to follow directions of therapist. They may persuade child to use tongue/lips in eating.

- *Medical*: Intercurrent illness may need treatment.
- *Psychiatric*: Diseases like attention deficit disorders may need to be managed time to time. Counseling and psychotherapy for older children may be needed for correction of behavioral abnormalities.
- *Special education*: Special education is determined by child's needs. Early intervention programs are useful. Individualized education program are needed. Socialization to promote self-concept development should be there.
- *Pharmacotherapy*:[6] Drugs like baclofen, diazepam, tizanidine, and dantrolene could be given to relieve spasticity. Intrathecal baclofen given via baclofen pump could be an option. Antianxiety drugs may relieve excessive emotions in patients with athetosis.
- *Botulinum toxin*: Botulinum toxin is produced by bacterium *Clostridium*. The drug blocks release of acetylcholine from cholinergic nerve terminals. Duration of effects lasts for 3–4 months. The adverse effects include muscle weakness. Allergic reactions are rare. Autonomic dysfunction such as occasional flu-like symptoms may occur.
- *Secondary complications*: Conditions like bowel and bladder problems, pneumonia, etc. need attention from time-to-time.

- *Nerve blocks*: Local nerve blocks to motor points of a muscle with a neurolytic agent (phenol solution) may relieve spasticity.

Prognosis

It is important to remember that cerebral palsy does not always cause profound disabilities. While one child with severe cerebral palsy might be unable to walk and need extensive, lifelong care, another with mild cerebral palsy might be only slightly awkward and require no special assistance. Supportive treatments, medications, and surgery can help many individuals improve their motor skills and ability to communicate with the world.

PREVENTION

Good antenatal and neonatal care is good preventive step. Early detection and timely advice could be important. Drugs are given for secondary care. Immunization and screening should be done timely and so is genetic counseling. Health education is important as well.

CONCLUSION

The brain damage that leads to cerebral palsy can also lead to other health issues, including vision, hearing, speech problems, and learning disabilities.

Common symptoms include lack of muscle coordination when performing voluntary movements (ataxia); stiff or tight muscles and exaggerated reflexes (spasticity); walking with one foot or leg dragging; walking on the toes, a crouched gait, or a "scissor" gait; and muscle tone that is either too stiff or too floppy. A small number of children have cerebral palsy as the result of brain damage in the first few months or years of life, brain infections such as bacterial meningitis or viral encephalitis, or head injury from a motor vehicle accident, a fall, or child abuse.

REFERENCES

1. Indian Academy of Pediatrics (2017). Neurology Chapter. [online] Available from https://www.iapindia.org/page.php?id=142. [Accessed May, 2018].
2. Abdel-Hamid HZ (2016). Cerebral palsy treatment and management. [online] Available from https://emedicine.medscape.com/article/1179555-treatment. [Accessed May, 2018].
3. WebMD (2017). What are the treatments for cerebral palsy? [online] Available from https://www.webmd.com/children/understanding-cerebral-palsy-treatment#1. [Accessed May, 2018].
4. National Health Trust Choices (2017). Cerebral palsy: Treatment. [online] Available from https://www.nhs.uk/conditions/cerebral-palsy/treatment/. [Accessed May, 2018].
5. Advancells (2017). Stem cell treatment for cerebral palsy. [online] Available from https://www.advancells.com/stem-cell-treatment-cerebral-palsy.php. [Accessed May, 2018].
6. Abdel-Hamid HZ (2016). Cerebral palsy medication. [online] Available from https://emedicine.medscape.com/article/1179555-medication. [Accessed May, 2018].

CHAPTER

19

Drug Treatment of Myositis/Myopathies

INTRODUCTION

Myopathies are diverse group of neurological disorders, with varied causes.

STATIN-INDUCED MYOPATHY

Statins are structural analogs of HMG-CoA reductase enzyme, the key enzyme for cholesterol biosynthesis. The drugs were first approved for the use in treatment of hypercholesterolemia about 30 years back. So far, they have been the most effective agents for reducing plasma cholesterol levels. They have been shown to be beneficial in prevention of primary and secondary coronary artery disease and reduce of mortality and morbidity. Overall, they are well-tolerated.

Statins are safe drugs. However, 2–3% statin users in randomized trials and about 10% of participants enrolled in prospective clinical studies develop myalgias. The rates of myositis are much lower and appear dose-dependent. Mean duration of statin therapy before onset of symptoms is 6 months. Mean duration of myalgias after stopping statin therapy is about 2 months.

Treatment

Significant symptoms may necessitate discontinuation of statin and most patients are asymptomatic but patients with creatine kinase (CK) values more than five times of their basal value need urgent statin discontinuation. Rhabdomyolysis is a rare entity. Once symptoms have resolved and the CK has returned to baseline, one can try pravastatin or fluvastatin with careful monitoring.

INFLAMMATORY MYOPATHIES

Examples include polymyositis, dermatomyositis, juvenile dermatomyositis, inclusion body myositis, myositis associated with collagen vascular disease, and myositis associated with malignancy. Inflammatory myopathies are rare heterogeneous group of acquired diseases characterized by inflammatory infiltrate of skeletal muscle. The condition is potentially treatable.

Inclusion Body Myositis

This is more common after age 50 years. Female predominance exists. Drugs and toxins causing inclusion body myositis include the following:

- Chloroquine
- Colchicine
- Corticosteroids
- Heroin
- Alcohol
- Fibrates/statins
- Zidovudine.

A variety of genetic and metabolic factors have also been blamed in addition to drugs and toxin. The disease presents with muscle weakness which is slow and progressive. Weakness in thighs, wrist, or fingers can occur. This may be accompanied by swallowing difficulty and patients have history of falls. Diagnosis is made by a combination of clinical examination, history, and muscle biopsy.

Treatment

The goal is to optimize muscle strength and function. Immunosuppressive drugs, e.g. azathioprine or corticosteroids are used in selected patients, especially with atypical presentation.[1] Physical, occupational, and speech therapy may be needed.

Polymyositis/Dermatomyositis

The heliotrope rash was first described in about 150 years back. Later, biopsy documented polymyositis in ruling out *Trichinella,* a common parasitic infection of the muscles. The condition has bimodal age distribution and occurs in older children and adults.

This condition involves progressive painless weakness, difficulty lifting above head/combing hair, difficulty arising from a low chair or toilet, and nasal regurgitation or choking when eating. Hoarseness and change in voice can occur. Ocular/facial muscle involvement is very uncommon. Fatigue, fever, and weight loss is common. Nonerosive inflammatory polyarthritis in rheumatoid-like distribution may occur as well. Raynaud's phenomenon, interstitial lung disease, cardiac abnormalities, and amyopathic dermatomyositis can be associated factors.

Diagnosis is made by a combination of clinical history, physical examination, electromyography, magnetic resonance imaging (MRI) of muscle to demonstrate inflammation, or muscle biopsy.[2,3]

Treatment

The condition has good response to corticosteroids. Drugs such as azathioprine may be used as steroid-sparing agent.[4] Also, rituximab is used in patients unresponsive to azathioprine. Physical, speech, and diet therapy is needed in support.

Prednisolone is the drug of choice in usual dose of 1 mg/kg. The dose is maintained for 2 months. Response to therapy should be assessed weekly or fortnightly.[2] Muscle strength and enzyme levels could be used as monitoring tool. Activity of daily living could be good guide as well. Prednisolone can be continued for 9–12 months in lowest possible dose.

Azathioprine is given in dose of 1.5–3 mg/kg/daily. The drug may not be effective for 3–4 months and one need to monitor its side effects as well [e.g. gastrointestinal (GI) side effects, bone marrow depression, and live function derangements].

Methotrexate in dose of 10–40 mg can be used either orally or subcutaneously or intramuscularly. Liver functions and blood cell count monitoring are needed. Patients unresponsive to above drugs may need cyclosporine, or tacrolimus. Mycophenolate, intravenous immunoglobulins, or cyclophosphamide has been tried. Plasmapheresis may be used when everything fails.

CONCLUSION

Many drugs or diseases can cause myopathies. Statins, though well tolerated are among the most common drugs. Identifying patients at risk, using low dose of drugs suspected of causing myopathies and prompt management of diseased cases can be the key.

REFERENCES

1. Lloyd TE (2017). Management of inclusion body myositis. [online] Available from https://www.uptodate.com/contents/management-of-inclusion-body-myositis. [Accessed May, 2018].
2. Hunter K, Lyon MG. Evaluation and management of polymyositis. Indian J Dermatol. 2012;57(5):371-4.
3. Choy EH, Isenberg DA. Treatment of dermatomyositis and polymyositis. Rheumatology. 2002;41(1):7-13.
4. John Hopkins Myositis Center (2017). Inclusion body myositis. [online] Available from https://www.hopkinsmyositis.org/myositis/inclusion-body-myositis/. [Accessed May, 2018].

CHAPTER

20

Drugs for Genetic Disorders

BACKGROUND

A genetic brain disorder is caused by a variation or a mutation in a gene and affects the development and function of the brain. Some genetic brain disorders are due to random gene mutations or mutations caused by environmental exposure, such as cigarette smoke. Other disorders are inherited, which means that a mutated gene or group of genes is passed down through a family. They can also be due to a combination of both genetic changes and other outside factors.

Some examples of genetic brain disorders include:

- Leukodystrophies
- Phenylketonuria
- Tay-Sachs disease
- Wilson disease.

INTRODUCTION TO GENETIC MEDICINE

The treatment of the more than 1,800 known monogenic hereditary disorders will depend on the development of "genetic medicines"—therapies that use the transfer of deoxyribonucleic acid (DNA) and/or ribonucleic acid (RNA) to modify gene expression to correct or compensate for an abnormal phenotype. Strategies include the use of somatic stem cells, gene transfer, RNA modification, and in the future, embryonic stem cells. Despite the efficacy of these technologies in treating experimental models of hereditary disorders, applying them successfully in the clinic is a great challenge, which will only be overcome by expending considerable intellectual and economic resources, and by solving societal concerns about modifications of the human genetic repertoire.

CERLIPONASE ALFA[1]

Cerliponase alfa is a hydrolytic lysosomal peptidase. Cerliponase alfa is indicated to slow the loss of ambulation in symptomatic pediatric patients 3 years of age and older with late infantile neuronal ceroid lipofuscinosis type 2, also known as tripeptidyl peptidase 1 deficiency.[1]

Cerliponase alfa, a proenzyme, and is taken up by target cells in the central nervous system (CNS), translocated to the lysosomes through the cation independent mannose-6-phosphate receptor. The drug hence is activated in the lysosome and the activated proteolytic form of rhTPP1 cleaves tripeptides from the N-terminus of proteins.[2]

The drug is supplied as an injection for intraventricular administration. Pretreatment of patients with antihistamines with or without antipyretics or corticosteroids is recommended prior to the start of infusion.

The recommended dosage is 300 mg administered once every other week as an intraventricular infusion followed by infusion of intraventricular electrolytes over approximately 4.5 hours. For complete information on preparation, specific intraventricular access device for use, and administration, see the full prescribing information. Adverse effects associated with the use of this drug are fever, electrocardiogram (ECG) abnormalities, gastrointestinal (GI) events, and occasional seizures. Cardiovascular side effects have occurred in some.[3]

ZINC ACETATE

Galzin has been approved for the treatment of Wilson's disease.[4] Wilson's disease is a potentially fatal inherited abnormality, occurring in one of 30,000 people, that causes excess copper to accumulate in the body, affecting the liver and the brain. Patients become ill as teenagers or as young adults with liver disease, often with neurologic symptoms. Galzin works by blocking absorption of copper from the intestine.

RUFINAMIDE[5]

Rufinamide is a triazole derivative. The exact mechanism of action is unknown. However, it is thought that rufinamide modulates the activity of sodium channels, and in particular, prolongation of the inactive state of the channel.

Rufinamide is specifically indicated for adjunctive treatment of seizures associated with Lennox-Gastaut syndrome in children 4 years and older and adults. Rufinamide is supplied as a 200 mg or 400 mg tablet for oral administration.

The recommended initial dose of the drug for pediatrics aged 4 years and older with Lennox-Gastaut syndrome is a daily dose of approximately 10 mg/kg/day administered in two equally divided doses. The dose should be increased by approximately 10 mg/kg increments every other day to a target dose of 45 mg/kg/day or 3,200 mg/kg/day, whichever is less, administered in two equally divided doses.

The recommended initial dose of the drug for adults with Lennox-Gastaut syndrome is a daily dose of 400–800 mg/day administered in two equally divided doses. The dose should be increased by 400–800 mg/day every 2 days until a maximum daily dose of 3,200 mg/day, administered in two equally divided doses is reached.[6]

VELAGLUCERASE ALFA[7]

Velaglucerase alfa is a human glucocerebrosidase (GCD) product developed using the company's proprietary gene activation technology. Gaucher disease, caused by deficiency of the enzyme GCD, results in accumulation of a toxic glycolipid substrate, called glucocerebroside. Velaglucerase alfa supplements or replaces beta-GCD, the enzyme that catalyzes the hydrolysis of glucocerebroside, reducing the amount of accumulated glucocerebroside and correcting the pathophysiology of Gaucher disease.

TALIGLUCERASE ALFA[8,9]

Taliglucerase alfa is a recombinant form of human GCD. It is a lysosomal glucocerebroside-specific enzyme that catalyzes the hydrolysis of glucocerebroside to glucose and ceramide. Subjects with Gaucher disease do not produce enough GCD, which leads to the accumulation of glucocerebroside in the spleen, liver, and bone marrow.

Gene Therapy

Gene therapy is a treatment or cure for disorders caused by mutated genes and is envolving therapy. It involves adding a normally functioning gene/s to restore normal function. Germline gene therapy would be the permanent transfer of a gene into sperm or egg cells. This way, the future generations can be cured of the disease. Somatic cell (body cell) gene therapy is ideally only the transfer of genes to the affected cells. Many diseases have been treated using experimental gene therapies, e.g. melanoma, severe combined immunodeficiencies (SCID), some forms of hereditary blindness and sickle cell anemia.

CONCLUSION

Genetic diseases are uncommon and are caused by abnormalities in DNA, which could be in the form of single base mutation (one gene) or in entire chromosomes. Treatment of genetic diseases is challenging and needs family counselling, supportive therapy and specific drugs as and when applicable.

REFERENCES

1. Biomarin (2017). Cerliponase alfa: Current clinical trials. [online] Available from http://www.biomarin.com/products/clinical-trials/cerliponase-alfa/. [Accessed May, 2018].
2. Biomarin (2017). Cerliponase alfa (BMN 190) for CLN2 disease. [online] Available from http://www.biomarin.com/products/pipeline/cerliponase-alfa-bmn-190-tpp1-for-cln2-disease/. [Accessed May, 2018].
3. Food and Drug Administration (FDA) (2017). Brineura (cerliponase alfa) injection. [online] Available from https://www.accessdata.fda.gov/drugsatfda_docs/nda/2017/761052Orig1s000TOC.cfm. [Accessed May, 2018].
4. WebMD (2017). Zinc acetate capsule. [online] Available from https://www.webmd.com/drugs/2/drug-75874/zinc-acetate-oral/details. [Accessed May, 2018].

5. Epilepsy Foundation (2017). Rufinamide. [online] Available from https://www.epilepsy.com/medications/rufinamide. [Accessed May, 2018].
6. Medscape (2017). Rufinamide (Rx). [online] Available from https://reference.medscape.com/drug/banzel-rufinamide-343010. [Accessed May, 2018].
7. Velaglucerase alfa for injection (2017). A review of velaglucerase alfa in Gaucher disease. [online] Available from https://www.vpriv.com/. [Accessed May, 2018].
8. Grabowski GA, Golembo M, Shaaltiel Y. Taliglucerase alfa: an enzyme replacement therapy using plant cell expression technology. Mol Genet Metab. 2014;112(1):1-8.
9. DrugBank (2017). Taliglucerase alfa. [online] Available from https://www.drugbank.ca/drugs/DB08876. [Accessed May, 2018].

CHAPTER

21

Adverse Drug Reactions in Neurological Practice

INTRODUCTION

Adverse drug reactions (ADRs), also known as "side effects", are a frequent cause of morbidity in hospital and the community. They have a significant cost both financially and in terms of quality of life.[1] Incidence of ADRs in a neurological unit is not very different from internal medicine. Since brain is affected commonly in ADRs, there is need to understand them well. The subject has been a matter of reviews, meta-analysis, and even books.

World Health Organization (WHO) defines an ADR as *a drug-related event that is noxious and unintended and occurs at doses used in humans for prophylaxis, diagnosis or therapy of disease, or for the modification of physiological function.*

However, this definition does not take into account the scenarios such as overdose, therapeutic failure, drug interactions, and drug withdrawal, which can also cause ADRs.

Healthcare professionals like physicians and neurologists play an important role in identifying, reporting, and preventing ADRs.[2]

CLASSIFICATION OF ADVERSE DRUG REACTIONS (TABLE 21.1)[1,3]

Adverse drug reactions can be classified into five categories:

1. Type A reactions (predictable)
2. Type B reactions (unpredictable)
3. Type C (continuous drug usage)
4. Type D (delayed)
5. Type E (end of dose).

Type A Reactions

Also known as augmented drug effects. These are usually dose dependent and largely predictable. Incidence and morbidity rates are high and mortality is low. For example, respiratory depression with opioid analgesia, cough with angiotensin converting enzyme (ACE) inhibitors, rivastigmine-induced nausea and vomiting, and withdrawal effects with benzodiazepines or alcohol.

Type B Reactions

This includes idiosyncratic, aberrant, or bizarre drug effects that are unrelated to the pharmacology of the drug. These types of reactions are usually unpredictable. Incidence and morbidity rates are low and mortality is high. Type B reactions are most commonly immunological (e.g. penicillin allergy).

FACTORS PREDISPOSING TO ADVERSE DRUG REACTIONS[4,5]

Factors that predispose to ADRs are many and varied and some are related only to specific disease/drug interactions, such as rash with amoxicillin in patients with glandular fever. However, the following factors are generally considered to increase patient risk:

TABLE 21.1: Classification of adverse drug reactions (ADRs).

Types of ADR	*Effect*	*Characteristic*	*Examples*
A	Dose-dependent ADR, occurs at higher dose, and may subside when lower than usual doses are used	Preventable	Nonsteroidal anti-inflammatory drug (NSAID)-induced ulcers Hypoglycemia induced by insulin injection
B	Genetically determined, unpredictable, no dose relationships, and rarely fatal too	Not preventable	Penicillin-induced anaphylaxis
C	Occurs after chronic treatment	Monitoring is needed	Glucocorticoid-induced osteoporosis
D	Occurs after years of treatment	Early signs of disease necessitate the drug withdrawal	Tardive dyskinesia induced by antipsychotics
E	Usually occur after the drug withdrawal	Opioid, benzodiazepine withdrawal could be serious	Slow tapering is needed
F	Drug failure	Repeated usage can lead to resistance	Persistence of throat infection despite beta-lactam antibiotic

- Age
- Renal impairment
- Hepatic impairment
- Frailty
- Polypharmacy

- Female gender
- Previous history of ADRs
- Genetics.

The first four factors predispose to type A reactions because they are determinants of drug toxicity, but the remaining factors predispose to type A or type B reactions.

REPORTING ADVERSE DRUG REACTIONS[6]

Most ADRs are not reported and this can lead to delays in identifying important drug reactions. The reasons for failure to report ADRs have been called the "seven deadly sins" (*see* below) which can lead to serious interference with imparting good quality healthcare. Pharmacists should attempt to address these and encourage their medical and nursing colleagues to report ADRs, in addition to sending in their own reports. Healthcare professionals' knowledge in the area of ADRs monitoring is deficient. This has been shown in a number of surveys done in Indian settings. The deficiency spans from MBBS students to higher healthcare professions. The National Pharmacovigilance Program of India suggests healthcare professionals to report the ADRs and anyone in the healthcare can report. Even patients are encouraged to report the ADRs to the concerned authorities. Suboptimal reporting may be due to several reasons (Table 21.2).[7]

DRUG INTERACTIONS

Drug interactions occur when the effect of a drug is altered by the coadministration of another drug, food, or drink. The outcome of any drug interaction could be beneficial or occasionally potentially harmful. Box 21.1 gives a list of common drug interactions.[8]

TABLE 21.2: "Seven deadly sins" leading to suboptimal care.[7]	
Complacency	A mistaken belief that only safe drugs are allowed onto the market and that these will not cause serious adverse drug reactions (ADRs). This is a mistaken behavior and can lead to serious reactions if the drugs are used indiscriminately.
Fear	Fear of involvement in litigation, or of a loss of patient confidence. This is gradually becoming prevalent in India.
Guilt	Guilt that the patient has been harmed by a prescribed treatment. However, this should not prevent the pharmacist to report the ADRs to the competent authority.
Ambition	Ambition to collect and publish a personal series of cases. This may lead to the unnecessary use of "challenge-re-challenge".
Ignorance	Ignorance of what should be reported or how to make a report. This is still a problem in India at large.
Shyness	A reluctance to report an effect for which there is only a suspicion that it is drug related. This may lead to gross underreporting.
Lethargy	This may include a lack of time or interest, inability to find a report card, etc.

Mechanism of Drug Interactions

Drug interactions can occur due to pharmacokinetic or pharmacodynamic mechanisms. Sometimes, the interaction can be caused by more than one mechanism, although usually one mechanism is more significant. The majority of interactions are caused by the mechanisms of absorption, distribution, metabolism, and excretion discussed here.

Pharmacokinetic Mechanisms

- *Absorption*: One drug will increase or decrease the absorption of another. Changes in the gastric

Box 21.1: Common drug interactions.[8]

- Tetracyclines absorption becomes reduced by milk products
- Absorption of warfarin may be reduced by griseofulvin
- Absorption of digoxin may be facilitated by metoclopramide
- Methotrexate may be displaced by aspirin
- Metabolism of theophylline may be blocked by ciprofloxacin
- Penicillin elimination is inhibited by probenecid
- Sildenafil given with nitrates can cause added hypotension.

pH affect the absorption of certain drugs, e.g. ketoconazole and itraconazole require an acidic environment to be absorbed, thus proton-pump inhibitors can reduce absorption and an acidic drink such as fruit juice or soft drinks will increase absorption. Most of drugs are absorbed from the upper part of the small intestine. Thus, changes in gut motility potentially affect absorption. Usually the total amount absorbed is unaffected, but the rate of absorption might be altered.

- *Distribution*: Some drugs are bound to proteins in the serum. Only unbound drug is active. Protein binding is a competitive effect so one drug can displace the other from protein-binding sites. This interaction is only an issue with highly protein-binding sites. This interaction is only significant if most of the drug remains in the plasma rather than being distributed into tissues. Displacement of drug from protein-binding sites often only causes a small "blip" in drug levels before equilibrium is restored (because the free drug is also now available for metabolism and excretion), but it could be significant for drugs with a narrow therapeutic index (e.g. warfarin).
- *Metabolism*: Induction or inhibition of the cytochrome P450 (CYP450) system lead to changes in drug levels. CYP450 represents a large group of isoenzymes; drugs are rarely metabolized by a single enzyme, although one usually predominates.

When only two drugs are involved, the effect is fairly easy to predict, even if each drug is likely to affect the metabolism of the other. However, if three or more drugs, all of which are inducers or inhibitors, are involved, the effect is almost impossible to predict and this type of combination should be avoided if possible. The full effects of enzyme induction and inhibition do not occur immediately.

- Enzyme induction takes about 2–3 weeks to develop and wear off.
- Enzyme inhibition takes only a few days.

Thus, it might be necessary to delay dose adjustment or therapeutic drug monitoring (TDM) until a few days (inhibition) or at least a week (induction) after starting or stopping the offending drug/s.

- *Excretion*: Some drugs interfere with excretion of other drugs. If both drugs are excreted by the same active transport system in the kidney tubule, the excretion of each drug is reduced by the other. This might be used as a beneficial effect. For example, probenecid has been used to prolong half-life of penicillin.

Pharmacodynamic Interactions

These types of interactions occur if the pharmacological effects of two drugs are additive or opposing:

- *Additive*: The desired or adverse effects of the two drugs are the same. This can be beneficial or potentially harmful. For example, increased sedation with alcohol plus hypnotics.
- *Synergism*: It is a form of additive effect. In this instance, the combination of the two drugs has a greater effect than just an additive effect. For example, ethambutol increases the effectiveness of other antitubercular drugs.
- *Antagonism*: At receptor level (e.g. a beta-blocker should be prescribed with caution to an asthmatic patient who

uses a beta-agonist inhaler) or because of opposing effects [e.g. the desired effects of diuretics could be, at least partly, opposed by fluid retention caused by nonsteroidal anti-inflammatory drugs (NSAIDs)].

Managing Drug Interactions[9]

If we keep the following things in mind, drug interactions could be managed easily. Managing drug interactions are important. Most of the drug interactions are either pharmacokinetic or pharmacodynamic. Some, however, have a pharmaceutical basis. Given here are useful tips:[9,10]

- Check whether or not the drug combination is new.
- If the patient has already been taking the drug combination, if they are able to tolerate it or not.
- If the interaction is potentially serious.
- The elderly are at greater risk of drug interactions, because of polypharmacy and impaired metabolism and excretion.
- Interactions can occur with nonprescription drugs also such as herbal or traditional medicines, over-the-counter medicines, and recreational drugs including alcohol, tobacco, etc.
- The potential interactions with high-risk drugs should always be checked. Like, enzyme inhibitors and inducers (e.g. erythromycin, rifampicin, phenytoin, and protease inhibitors), and drugs with narrow therapeutic index (e.g. warfarin, digoxin, lithium, phenytoin, theophylline, and gentamicin).

CONCLUSION

Adverse drug reaction (ADR) is a noxious and unintended response to a drug that occurs at normal therapeutic doses used in humans for prevention, diagnosis, or treatment of disease.[10] Side effect on the other hand is any unintended effect of a pharmaceutical product occurring at normal therapeutic doses and is related to its pharmacological properties. Such effects may be well-known and even expected and require little or no change in patient management. Serious adverse effect is any untoward medical occurrence that occurs at any dose and results in death, requires hospital admission or prolonged hospital stay, results in persistent or significant disability, or is life-threatening.

Pharmacovigilance is the science and activities relating to the detection, assessment, understanding and prevention of adverse effects or any other drug-related problem. World Health Organization established its programme for International Drug Monitoring in response to the thalidomide disaster (1961) center for spontanneous ADR monitoring in Uppsala, Sweden. Drugs used in neurology and psychiatry practice commonly cause adverse drug reactions hence need regular monitoring.

REFERENCES

1. Dhikav V, Singh S, Anand KS (2004). Adverse drug reaction monitoring in India. [online] Available from http://medind.nic.in/jac/t04/i1/jact04i1p27.pdf. [Accessed May, 2018].
2. Khan SA, Goyal C, Chandel N, et al. Knowledge, attitudes, practice of doctors to adverse drug reaction reporting in a teaching hospital in India: An observational study. J Nat Sci Biol Med. 2013;4(1):191-6.
3. News Roundup (2004). Patient and adverse drug reactions monitoring in India. [online] Available from https://www.bmj.com/rapid-response/2011/10/30/patients-and-adverse-drug-reactions-monitoring-india. [Accessed May, 2018].
4. World Health Organization (WHO) (2017). Adverse drug reactions monitoring. [online] Available from http://www.who.int/medicines/areas/quality_safety/safety_efficacy/advdrugreactions/en/. [Accessed May, 2018].

5. Tanzania Foods and Drug Authority (TFDA) (2006). Guidelines for monitoring and reporting adverse drug reactions (ADRs). [online] Available from http://apps.who.int/medicinedocs/documents/s18571en/s18571en.pdf. [Accessed May, 2018].
6. Adverse Drug Reactions Database (2017). Overview of adverse drug reactions database. [online] Available from http://www.adr-database.com/What%20are%20ADRs.html. [Accessed May, 2018].
7. Marsh DE (2017). Overview of adverse drug reactions (side effects; adverse effects). [online] Available from https://www.merckmanuals.com/home/drugs/adverse-drug-reactions/overview-of-adverse-drug-reactions. [Accessed May, 2018].
8. Government of Canada (2017). Consultation: mandatory reporting of serious adverse drug reactions and medical device incidents. [online] Available from https://www.canada.ca/en/health-canada/programs/consultation-reporting-serious-adverse-drug-reactions-medical-device-incidents.html. [Accessed May, 2018].
9. Health Sciences Authority (2017). Adverse drug reaction news bulletin. [online] Available from http://www.hsa.gov.sg/content/hsa/en/Health_Products_Regulation/Safety_Information_and_Product_Recalls/Adverse_Drug_Reaction_News_Bulletin.html. [Accessed May, 2018].
10. ADRs (2017). Reporting suspected adverse drug reactions. [online] Available from https://www.google.co.in/search?q=adverse+drug+reactions+WHO&ei=uHcuWtPRNcGBvwT774_IDw&start=10&sa=N&biw=1242&bih=611. [Accessed May, 2018].

CHAPTER

22

Anticancers in Neurology

BRAIN TUMORS

Brain tumors are not uncommon with an incidence of 8–25/100,000. It is important to know that it could be an important cause of the death. It could be primary or metastasis which includes one-fourth of all tumors.

Etiology

There seems to be genetical predisposition. Hereditary factors, e.g. von Recklinghausen disease, tuberous sclerosis play roles. Viral infections like Epstein-Barr virus may play a role in etiology of primary brain lymphoma. Likewise, environmental factors such as pesticides, chemicals also play important roles. Tumors could be primary or secondaries (Box 22.1).

Secondary Tumors

These tumors cells reach the brain via the bloodstream. Prognosis of brain tumors is variable and varies as per

BOX 22.1: Secondaries tumors in brain.

- Lung
- Breast
- Kidneys
- Malignant melanoma
- Gastrointestinal tract (GIT)
- Thyroid gland
- Gynecologic tumors
- Prostate
- Originate from malignant tumors located primarily in other organs
- *Skin:* Malignant melanoma
- *Kidney:* Hypernephroma
- *Breast:* Breast carcinoma
- *Colon:* Colon carcinoma.

histological structures. Biopsy showing cell atypical shapes and sizes, mitotic activity, and abnormal mitosis may have bad prognosis. Localization also has an important role to play in predicting prognosis, e.g. benign tumors in brainstem or deep structures have a bad prognosis.

Meningioma

This is a common primary tumor of the brain accounting for 30% of brain tumors and is treatable. Localization is on the hemispheres convexity, parasagittal, or olfactorius, sella turcica, cerebello-pontine, tentorium, etc. It is usually benign. Bone protrusion or hyperostosis may occur specially in frontal bones. Parasagittal meningioma may be associated with monoparesis of contralateral lower extremity or paraparesis. Near bulbus olfactorius, it may be associated with unilateral anosmia. In the proximity of optic nerve, exophthalmos, or monocular blindness, ipsilateral mydriasis with absent fundal reflex. Near sphenoidal bone wings, it may be associated with epileptic seizures, lesion of cranial nerves. Cerebello-pontine meningiomas are associated with loss of hearing, dizziness, and Bell's palsy.[1] Surgery is the primary form of treatment but several drug treatments are being explored: Hydroxyurea, mifepristone (progesterone antagonist), somatostatin analogs, octreotide, everolimus, and vascular endothelial growth factor (VEGF) blocker, e.g. imatinib.[1]

Paraneoplastic Syndrome

Sometimes, the symptoms of paraneoplastic syndromes are present even before the diagnosis of a malignancy (Box 22.2). A total of about 10% patients with tumors may have paraneoplastic syndrome. Antibodies against neuronal structures (anti Yo, anti Hu, and anti Ri) may be present. All parts of nervous system may be involved, e.g. central, peripheral, neuromuscular junction, or muscles.

Treatment

A variety of medical treatment modalities, including chemotherapy and radiotherapy, are used alone or in combination with surgical resection. Supportive care includes steroids, anticonvulsant drugs, etc.

ANTICANCER DRUGS IN NEUROLOGY

Anticancer drugs in brain tumors can be classified according to chemical structure and resource of the drug,

Box 22.2: Causes of paraneoplastic syndromes.

- Small cell lung carcinoma
- Breast carcinoma
- Ovarial carcinoma
- Hodgkin's lymphoma
- Thymoma
- Neuroblastoma
- Prostatic carcinoma.

molecular mechanisms of anticancer action, according to the cycle, or phase specificity of the drug.

General mechanisms include block of nucleic acid material, e.g. [deoxyribonucleic acid (DNA), ribonucleic acid (RNA)] biosynthesis. They can also directly destroy DNA and inhibit DNA reproduction. They may interfere transcription and block RNA synthesis or interfere protein synthesis and function.

Additionally several anticancer drugs act by influencing hormone homeostasis. Examples include antimetabolites, *folic acid antagonist, or* inhibit dihydrofolate reductase (methotrexate). *Pyrimidine antagonist such as fluorouracil* inhibits thymidylate synthase inhibitors are used in a variety of cancers. They inhibit DNA polymerase (cytarabine).

Purine antagonists inhibit interconversion of purine nucleotide mercaptopurine. Hydroxyurea has been tried in meningioma and associated with neuropathy. Protein synthesis inhibitors, e.g. anticancer antibiotics are used commonly. Antitubulins, e.g. vinca alkaloids and taxanes, interferes the function of ribosomes and produce mitotic arrest. Harringtonines and L-asparaginase influence amino acid supply.

Inhibition of RNA synthesis is a prominent mechanism of anticancer antibiotics. They bind with DNA to block RNA production. Doxorubicin can influence the structure and function of DNA.

ALKYLATING AGENTS

Drugs like mechlorethamine, cyclophosphamide, and thiotepa are commonly used alkylating agents.

Mechanism of Action

Alkylating agents are nitrogen mustards that inhibit cell reproduction by binding irreversibly with the nucleic acids (DNA). The specific type of chemical bonding involved is *alkylation*. After alkylation, DNA is unable to replicate and therefore can no longer synthesize proteins and other essential cell metabolites. Consequently, cell reproduction is inhibited and the cell eventually dies from the inability to maintain its metabolic functions.

Anticancer Drug Resistance

Membrane transport may be decreased. The drug may be bound by glutathione (GSH) via GSH S-transferase or metallothioneins in the cytoplasm and inactivated. The drug may be metabolized to inactive species.

Side Effects

Myelosuppression is the dose-limiting adverse effect for alkylating agents. Nausea and vomiting are common as are teratogenesis and gonadal atrophy, although in the latter cases these are variable, according to the drug, its schedule, and route of administration. Treatment also carries a major risk of leukemogenesis and carcinogenesis.

Cyclophosphamide

Cyclophosphamide is used in the treatment of chronic lymphocytic leukemia, non-Hodgkin's lymphomas, breast and ovarian cancer, and a variety of other cancers. It is also a potent immunosuppressant; it is used in the management of rheumatoid disorders and autoimmune nephritis. In neurology, it is used for multiple sclerosis and transverse myelitis.[2] Adverse effects include alopecia, nausea, vomiting, myelosuppression, and hemorrhagic cystitis.

Nitrosoureas

Examples include carmustine, lomustine, semustine, etc. Pharmacokinetically, nitrosoureas are highly lipophilic and reach cerebrospinal fluid concentrations that are about 30% of plasma concentrations. Because of their excellent central nervous system (CNS) penetration, carmustine and lomustine have been used to treat brain tumors since long.

Carmustine must be injected intravenously because it is highly reactive. It disappears very rapidly from the blood, the activity of mustine lasts only a few minutes. It is used commonly in brain cancers.[3,4] The main indication for mustine is in treatment of Hodgkin's disease and lymphomas, but it may also be useful in other malignancies as well.

Melphalan

Melphalan is a nitrogen mustard that is primarily used to treat multiple myeloma (plasma cell myeloma), breast cancer, and ovarian cancer. The drug has been associated with encephalopathy or brachial plexus neuritis.

ANTIMETABOLITES

Antimetabolites are S phase-specific drugs that are structural analogs of essential metabolites and that interfere with DNA synthesis. Myelosuppression is the dose-limiting toxicity for all drugs in this class.

Methotrexate[5,6]

The structures of methotrexate and folic acid are similar and are actively transported into mammalian cells. Methotrexate works by inhibiting dihydrofolate reductase, the enzyme that normally converts dietary folate to the tetrahydrofolate form required for thymidine and purine synthesis.

Methotrexate is used in the treatment of choriocarcinoma, a trophoblastic tumor, was the first demonstration of curative chemotherapy. It is especially effective for treating acute lymphocytic leukemia and for treating the meningeal metastases of a wide range of tumors.

Main side effect of methotrexate is myelosuppressive, producing severe leukopenia, bone marrow aplasia, and thrombocytopenia. This agent may produce severe gastrointestinal disturbances. Renal toxicity may occur because of precipitation of crystals. In neurology, the drug is used in myasthenia gravis and multiple sclerosis.[6]

ANTIESTROGEN

Tamoxifen[7]

Tamoxifen is the drug of choice in postmenopausal women with or recovering from metastatic breast cancer. It is most effective in patients who have estrogen receptor-positive tumors. Tamoxifen is also used as adjunctive therapy to oophorectomy to leuprolide or goserelin in premenopausal women with estrogen receptor-positive tumors. Cerebral venous sinus thrombosis is recognized as a risk factor of tamoxifen.[7]

Androgens

Androgen activity in breast cancer is similar to that of estrogens, perhaps for the same mechanistic reasons. Virilizing effects and hepatic toxicity make them unacceptable to most patients. Fluoxymesterone is the most widely used agent. Danazol has use in hematology in aplastic anemia and congenital anemias. A variety of neurological disorders like manic episodes, or aggression have been reported as side effects.[8]

Glucocorticoids

They are integral components of curative therapy for acute lymphoblastic leukemia, non-Hodgkin's lymphoma, and Hodgkin's disease. Glucocorticoids have essential roles in the prevention of allergic reaction, emesis control, relief of intracranial hypertension or spinal cord compression in neurologic complications, and pain relief. Optic neuritis, multiple sclerosis are other common clinical uses of glucocorticoids in neurology clinical medicine.[9]

Resistance to Anticancers

De Novo Resistance

De novo resistance can be de novo genetic (i.e. the cells are initially inherently resistant), or can arise because drugs are unable to reach the target cells because of permeability barriers such as the blood-brain barrier.

Acquired Resistance

Acquired drug resistance may result from genomic mutations, such as the induction or deletion of enzymes involved in drug inactivation or drug activation, respectively.

Multidrug Resistance

P-glycoprotein transports many naturally occurring drugs out of neoplastic cells, and its induction may lead to multidrug resistance. As scientific understanding of the mechanisms of drug resistance increases, new treatments may be developed to counteract resistance.

Common Side Effects

The most common toxicities of antineoplastic drugs result from inhibition of cell replication in the bone marrow, gastrointestinal epithelium, and hair follicles. Many antineoplastic drugs also stimulate the chemoreceptor trigger zone in the medulla and thereby elicit nausea and vomiting.

CONCLUSION

Neurological cancers are treated by a group of multidisciplinary team/s. Team includes neurologists, psychiatrists, neuro-oncologists, physicians, assistants, oncology nurses, social workers, pharmacists, counselors, dietitians, and others.

The size, type, and grade of the tumor are main concerns. Additionally, whether the tumor is putting pressure on vital parts of the brain is an important issue. If the tumor has spread to other parts of the CNS or body, possible side effects and the patient's preferences and overall health are important indicators.

Some types of brain tumors grow rapidly, e.g. glioblastoma and others are slowly growing (e.g. meningioma). Treatment options include surgery, radiation therapy, and chemotherapy. Tumor care plan may also include treatment for symptoms and side effects of the drugs or any other treatment/s.

REFERENCES

1. American Brain Tumor Association (2017). Meningioma. [online] Available from http://www.abta.org/secure/meningioma-brochure.pdf. [Accessed May, 2018].
2. Awad A, Stüve O. Cyclophosphamide in multiple sclerosis: scientific rationale, history and novel treatment paradigms. Ther Adv Neurol Disord. 2009;2(6):50-61.
3. Levačić D, Nochlin D, Steineke T, et al (2012). Management of malignant meningiomas. [online] Available from http://cdn.intechopen.com/pdfs/30673.pdf. [Accessed May, 2018].
4. Cancer Research (2017). Cancer: General features and its treatment. [online] Available from https://www.cancerresearchuk.org/about-cancer/cancer-in-general/treatment/cancer-drugs/drugs/carmustine. [Accessed May, 2018].

5. Neurology (2017). Neuromuscular disease: Methotrexate has no steroid-sparing effect in patients with generalized myasthenia gravis. [online] Available from https://www.nature.com/articles/nrneurol.2016.103. [Accessed May, 2018].
6. Neurology Lounge (2016). What is the startling research unsettling the treatment of myasthenia gravis? [online] Available from https://theneurologylounge.com/tag/methotrexate/. [Accessed May, 2018].
7. Masjuan J, Pardo J, Callejo JM, et al. Tamoxifen: a new risk factor for cerebral sinus thrombosis. Neurology. 2004;62(2):334-5.
8. Christiansen K, Knussmann R. Androgen levels and components of aggressive behavior in men. Horm Behav. 1987;21(2):170-80.
9. Sivakumar MR (2017). Corticosteroids in neurology. [online] Available from http://www.thamburaj.com/corticosteroids_in_neurology.htm. [Accessed May, 2018].

CHAPTER

23

Drug-induced Neurological Disorders

INTRODUCTION

Drugs used in medicine are an important reversible cause of common neurological disorders.[1] Though several mechanisms exist for drug-induced neurological diseases but mitochondrial toxicity is an important mechanism.[2] Early recognition of drug-induced neurological disorders (DINDs) and drug withdrawal can prevent irreversible damage.

There are several reasons for DINDs, e.g. drug interactions can increase the toxicity of single agents. Such problems can occur at initiation, during sudden withdrawal of therapy (e.g. tramadol withdrawal seizures), and after many months or years of therapy (e.g. valproate encephalopathy). Treatment is primarily concerned with controlled withdrawal, but toxic levels may necessitate hemodialysis or hemofiltration (e.g. lithium), specific neutralizing therapies (e.g. antibody fragments in digoxin overdose), or symptomatic treatments. Several individual examples are given here.

SEIZURES[1]

Seizures may be caused by antipsychotics, antidepressants, antineoplastic agents (alkylators, antimetabolites, vinca alkaloids, ifosfamide, and cisplatin), penicillins, cephalosporins, quinolones, antimalarials, aminophylline, and allopurinol. They are frequently observed in drug-induced encephalopathy. Commonly encountered drugs in neurology leading to seizures are given in Box 23.1.

Other less frequently reported drugs which may induce seizures include opioids, baclofen, digoxin, dopaminergic agents, thyroxine, and ondansetron in overdose.

STROKE

Drug-induced cerebrovascular disease may be related to antihypertensives and arrhythmogenic agents that can cause focal ischemia, particularly in the elderly, with right shifted autoregulation and underlying atherosclerotic arterial stenoses. Cancer chemotherapy may cause thromboembolism, hemorrhage, vasospasm, or vasculitis; probably because of the synergistic actions of factors secreted by the tumor or products of tumor lysis. Common causes of drug-induced seizures in neurological/psychiatric practice are given here (Boxes 23.1 and 23.2).

HEADACHE[3-5]

Drugs that cause headache usually do so by exacerbating preexisting migraine, tension headache, or chronic daily headache. Analgesics, including those used to treat headache, may also cause the analgesic overuse syndrome seen most commonly in frequent use of opiate-based analgesia. Drugs used in the treatment of other medical conditions which can cause headache include antidepressants, H1 and H2 blockers, anti-fungals, antihypertensives, beta-blockers, sulfonamides,

Box 23.1: Common drugs responsible for seizures in neurology/ psychiatry.

- Bupropion
- Tramadol
- Diphenhydramine
- Venlafaxine.

Box 23.2: Drug-induced seizures in neurological/psychiatric practice.

- Street drugs
- Sumatriptan
- Oral anticoagulants
- Antihypertensives
- Thrombolytics.

intravenous immunoglobulin, and oral contraceptive pills (Box 23.3).

Visual disturbance and papilloedema associated with drug-induced headache is idiopathic intracranial hypertension. Tetracyclines, retinoids, corticosteroids, estrogen receptor agonists and antagonists, nonsteroidal anti-inflammatory drugs, growth hormone, cimetidine, nalidixic acid, trimethoprim-sulfamethoxazole, amiodarone, and lithium are all associated with idiopathic hypertension of intracranial area.

ENCEPHALOPATHY

Morphine and propofol were historically first drugs associated with drug-induced encephalopathy.[6] After this, a variety of drugs such as antidepressants, antiepileptic, and antibiotics, etc. have been associated. Drugs that cause encephalopathy and coma do so either by inducing metabolic disturbances (e.g. hepatic, hypoglycemic, hyponatremic, or uremic encephalopathy) or by direct central nervous system toxicity (antiepileptics, beta-lactam antibiotics, etc.). Drug-induced coma most commonly

Box 23.3: Drug-induced headache in neurological/psychiatric practice.

- Medication overuse [nonsteroidal anti-inflammatory drug (NSAID) overuse]
- Nitrates
- Benzodiazepine withdrawal.

occurs at toxic serum concentrations of drug, typically after overdose [e.g. tricyclic antidepressants (TCAs), opiates, benzodiazepines, and antiepileptics]. Posterior reversible leukoencephalopathy, often associated with seizures and hypertension occurs in transplant patients treated with immunosuppressives, e.g. ciclosporin or tacrolimus. Other drugs known to cause posterior reversible encephalopathy include antivirals (e.g. acyclovir), antifungal (e.g. amphotericin), anticancers (e.g. cisplatin, cytarabine, ifosfamide, and methotrexate, etc.).

DEMENTIA[7,8]

Dementia may be caused by several drugs, e.g. anticholinergics, antihypertensives, antiepileptics, antipsychotics with anticholinergic activity, benzodiazepines, corticosteroids, and interferons can all cause a reversible condition resembling dementia. Drug-induced dementia is a diagnosis of exclusion.

EXTRAPYRAMIDAL DISORDERS[9]

Drug-induced extrapyramidal side effects traditionally occur due to D2 blockers, e.g. phenothiazines, haloperidol. Other drugs have been associated with extrapyramidal side effects as well, e.g. TCAs, antiemetics like metoclopramide, and antipsychotic, e.g. lithium. Major types of extrapyramidal symptoms are given here in Box 23.4.

The first generation or older antipsychotics may cause significant extrapyramidal side effects, more so than the second-generation antipsychotic agents.

Box 23.4: Major types of extrapyramidal symptoms.

- Dystonia
- Parkinsonism
- Akathisia
- Tardive dyskinesia.

Risperidone and ziprasidone are more likely to cause extrapyramidal side effects amongst second-generation antipsychotic agents.

Acute dystonia and oculogyric crisis is caused by antipsychotics, TCAs, antiepileptic drugs (AEDs), and metoclopramide. It occurs usually within 48 hours of initiation of the medication. The condition involves severe muscle contractions and can be painful. Acute muscular dystonia is accompanied by odd posturing and strange facial expressions.

Parkinson's disease occurs after 3 or more weeks of treatment. The condition is characterized by cogwheeling rigidity, tremors, rhythmic oscillations of the legs, and pill rolling movement of the fingers.

Akathisia occurs after 3 or more weeks of treatment. The condition is experienced as desire or need to move. In severe cases, there can be an inability to sit idle.

Choreoathetosis is seen with neuroleptics and oral contraceptives. TCAs and antipsychotics can both cause restless leg syndrome, while dextroamphetamine, methylphenidate, and haloperidol can cause motor tics.

Management

Drug withdrawal is the first step but acute symptomatic treatment is also often required [e.g. intravenous (IV) diphenhydramine/IV diazepam/lorazepam. Tardive dyskinesia, which develops after prolonged treatment with antipsychotics can even be irreversible. It may be prevented by concomitant treatment with vitamin E but stopping D2 blockers is needed. One can start clozapine or tetrabenazine. Sulpiride could be useful as well. Patients may complain of akathisia when treated with antipsychotics, and can be propranolol.

TREMORS[10]

Sodium valproate, lithium are common drugs. Patients taking beta-agonists for treatment of asthma often experience tremors. Additionally, those taking theophylline often have tremulous hands. Drugs like cyclosporine and tacrolimus too can cause tremors. Beta-blockers are used for treatment. However, in asthma, they are avoided and condition can respond to dosage alterations.

MYOCLONUS AND NYSTAGMUS[11,12]

Drugs like TCAs, lithium, antipsychotics, levodopa, and dopamine agonists can cause myoclonus. Myoclonus persisting after drug withdrawal or reduction can be treated with clonazepam, or sodium valproate, piracetam or levetiracetam.

The most common drug-induced neurological disease of eye movements is nystagmus and is caused by benzodiazepines, antiepileptics like phenytoin, monoamine oxidase inhibitors, salicylates, lithium, or fenfluramine, etc. Overdose of phenytoin may be responsible as well in first few days. Benzodiazepines and lithium have been associated with internuclear ophthalmoplegia and needs to differentiate this from multiple sclerosis.

NEUROPATHY[13]

Anticancers such as cytosine arabinoside, ciclosporin, and ganciclovir can all induce abducens palsies. Early withdrawal of therapy is essential to ensure recovery.

Drugs that induce subacute myelo-optico-neuropathy are thought to do so by depleting vitamins (particularly B vitamins and vitamin E) or by inhibiting their intracellular cofactors (copper and zinc dependent). Drug-induced neuropathies can be demyelinating, axonal, or mixed with elements of axonal loss and demyelination. B vitamins, glutathione, and zinc supplements are often used in treatment and the offending agent needs to be discontinued. Neuropathy is a common side effect of antiretroviral drugs. Myopathy can occur with zidovudine. Neuropsychiatric reactions occur commonly to efavirenz. Immune inflammatory syndrome occurs due to use of highly active antiretroviral therapy in human immunodeficiency virus (HIV). Monoclonal antibodies can be the cause of neurological disorders as well.

CONCLUSION

The term neurologic side effect is commonly used to describe a new drug-induced neurologic syndrome and/or disorder. Physicians may not routinely anticipate or recognize these new conditions caused by commonly used drugs. Changes in the central nervous system (brain, spinal cord) or peripheral nerves can cause a wide variety of symptoms, including loss of coordination and muscle strength, numbness, loss of consciousness, seizures, and paralysis. Even drugs used in psychiatric conditions like insomnia, anxiety, depression can simulate neurological conditions and *vice versa*. Drugs should be kept in differential diagnosis of unexplained psychiatric/neurological symptoms.

REFERENCES

1. Zagaria MA (2010). Common causes of drug-induced seizures. [online] Available from https://www.uspharmacist.com/article/common-causes-of-drug-induced-seizures. [Accessed May, 2018].

2. Healthy.Net (2017). Drugs causing stroke. [online] Available from http://www.healthy.net/scr/article.aspx?Id=2858. [Accessed May, 2018].
3. Up-To-Date (2017). Drugs-induced headache. [online] Available from https://www.uptodate.com/contents/search?search=Drug-Induced%20Headache. [Accessed May, 2018].
4. Diener HC, Wilkinson M (1988). Drug-induced headache. [online] Available from http://www.springer.com/in/book/9783642733291. [Accessed May, 2018].
5. WebMD (2017). Medicines that can cause headaches. [online] Available from https://www.webmd.com/migraines-headaches/medication-headaches#1. [Accessed May, 2018].
6. Hansen L (2012). Drug-induced encephalopathy. [online] Available from https://www.intechopen.com/books/miscellanea-on-encephalopathies-a-second-look/drug-induced-encephalopathy. [Accessed May, 2018].
7. Dementia.org (2017). Genetics and dementia: what are the risk factors? [online] Available from https://www.dementia.org/genetics-and-dementia-what-are-the-risk-factors. [Accessed May, 2018].
8. Moore AR, O'Keefee ST. Drug-induced cognitive impairment in the elderly. Drugs Aging. 1999;15(1):15-28.
9. Owens DG (2014). A guide to the extrapyramidal side-effects of antipsychotic drugs. [online] Available from http://bjp.rcpsych.org/content/206/5/437. [Accessed May, 2018].
10. Morgan JC, Sethi KD. Drug-induced tremors. Lancet. 2005;4(12):866-76.
11. Jiménez-Jiménez FJ, Puertas I, de Toledo-Heras M. Drug-induced myoclonus: frequency, mechanism and management. CNS Drugs. 2004;18(2):93-104.
12. Bardorf CM (2017). Acquired nystagmus. [online] Available from https://emedicine.medscape.com/article/1199177-overview. [Accessed May, 2018].
13. Argov Z, Mastaglia FL. Drug-induced peripheral neuropathies. Br Med J. 1979;1(6164):663-6.

Index

Page numbers followed by *b* refer to box, *f* refer to figure, *fc* refer to flowchart, and *t* refer to table

C

D

I

J

K

L

M

N

O

P

Q

R

S

T

U

V

W

Z